Mind Body Fitness

Mind Body Fitness

HEALING FOR THE MIND AND BODY

Z Altug, PT, DPT, MS, CSCS

Physical Therapist / Assistant Professor
West Coast University
Los Angeles, California

CreateSpace
4900 Lacross Road
North Charleston, SC 29406
www.createspace.com

ISBN-13: 9781540357519
ISBN-10: 1540357511
Library of Congress Control Number: 2016919073
CreateSpace Independent Publishing Platform
North Charleston, South Carolina

Disclaimer

This book is for educational purposes and is not a substitute for medical advice, diagnosis, or treatment. All reasonable effort has been made to ensure the accuracy of the information in this book. However, due to ongoing research and discoveries, the information in this book may not reflect the latest standards, developments, or treatments.

Readers who have questions about a particular condition or treatment should consult with a physician or healthcare provider. The author shall not be liable for any damages allegedly arising from the information in this book. The author is also not responsible for errors or omissions or for any consequences from the application of the information in this book and makes no warranty, expressed or implied, with respect to the currency, completeness, or accuracy of the contents of the publication.

As with all health and fitness programs, the reader should get a physician's approval before beginning an exercise, nutrition, or any other self-help routine. Any practice or guideline described in this book should be applied by the reader in conjunction with the advice of his or her healthcare provider and/or fitness professional.

Remember to follow these four golden rules: 1) Do no harm. 2) If you are in doubt about something in this book, check it out with your healthcare provider and/or fitness professional. 3) Start slowly and progress gradually. 4) And, finally, listen to your mind and body signals.

All trademarks, trade names, model names and numbers, and any other designations referred to herein are the property of their respective owners and are used solely for identification purposes.

To Mom and Dad for preparing me for my journey in life

About the Author

Z Altug, PT, DPT, MS, CSCS, is a licensed physical therapist and performance specialist with more than 27 years of experience in his field. He currently works as an assistant professor at West Coast University in Los Angeles and as a private consultant. Z previously worked at the UCLA Medical Center outpatient rehabilitation department for 12 years. He graduated from the University of Pittsburgh with a bachelor of science degree in physical therapy and obtained his master of science degree in sport and exercise studies and a bachelor of science degree in physical education from West Virginia University. Z also completed a transitional doctorate degree in physical therapy (DPT) from the College of St. Scholastica in Duluth, Minnesota, and is a long-standing member of the American Physical Therapy Association, California Physical Therapy Association, and National Strength and Conditioning Association.

Z is certified by the National Strength and Conditioning Association (NSCA) as a certified strength and conditioning specialist (CSCS) and personal trainer (NSCA-CPT). Additionally, he was twice certified by USA Track & Field as a level 1 coach and twice by USA Weightlifting as a level 1 sport performance coach. Z also has completed workshops and classes in yoga, tai chi, qigong, the Pilates method, the Feldenkrais Method, and the Alexander Technique to further expand his knowledge of body movement.

Beyond sharing his knowledge and experience with personal clients, Z extends his reach through writing. Z coauthored *Patalosh: The Time Travelers* (CreateSpace, 2015), *2012 Healthy Lifestyle Wall and Engagement Calendars* (TF Publishing, 2011), *The Anti-Aging Fitness Prescription* (Hatherleigh Press, 2006), and the *Manual of Clinical Exercise Testing, Prescription and Rehabilitation* (Appleton & Lange, 1993) and authored

Sustainable Fitness: A Practical Guide to Health, Healing, and Wellness (CreateSpace, 2016).

Z enjoys participating in a variety of sports, learning about astronomy, and discussing new projects with his two rowdy cats at his home in Los Angeles.

For further information about Z, see www.linkedin.com/in/zaltug and www.facebook.com/zaltugfitness.

Acknowledgments

thank Dad, an internal medicine specialist, for having shared his medical knowledge with me.

I thank Mom for encouraging me to take time to appreciate art, music, dance, poetry, and literature from different cultures.

Preface

Dear Reader,

Mind Body Fitness: Healing for the Mind and Body can be used by individuals looking for simple tips and guidelines to supplement the advice provided by their healthcare professionals. The purpose of this book is to provide a practical foundation which bridges the gap between Eastern and Western movement systems and practices. The book is written in a format that largely uses bullet-points, checklists, tables, charts, and boxes to help readers easily extract and use the information.

I wish you good health and happiness.

Z Altug, PT, DPT, MS, CSCS
Los Angeles, CA

Contents

Exercise Index

PART 1
Healing Faster

The following are some simple tips to help you heal faster after injury, surgery, or illness:

Ask Your Doctor About Preoperative Training
There is some evidence that getting in shape before surgery can help you recover faster and reduce complications after surgery (dos Santos Alves et al. 2014; Humphrey et al. 2015). Consider this as the "better in, better out" approach (Hoogeboom et al. 2014). Ask your doctor if you would benefit from preoperative physical therapy and fitness training. Before your surgery it is also a good time to quit smoking, limit alcohol, improve your diet, establish better sleep patterns, and learn to control your stress levels. You can also have a discussion with your healthcare provider about how you can prepare your home for after surgery, such as installing grab bars in the shower, or purchasing a raised toilet seat or safety rails around the toilet for assistance in sitting and standing.

Ask Your Doctor or Therapist
BEMER (Bio-Electro-Magnetic-Energy-Regulation) is a medical device which increases microcirculation and helps reduce pain and supports the body's own self-healing and regeneration processes. For more information about BEMER, refer to the BEMER group website at www.bemergroup.com.

A study by Gyulai et al. (2015) shows that "BEMER physical vascular therapy reduced pain and fatigue in the short term in patients with chronic low back pain, while long-term therapy appears to be beneficial in patients with osteoarthritis of knee."

Another study by Piatkowski et al. (2009) shows "a beneficial effect of BEMER intervention on multiple sclerosis (MS) fatigue."

Brighten Your Home
Pull back the curtains, and open the shades. Bring more natural outdoor light into your home during the day to help you heal (Beauchemin et al. 1996, 1998).

Care for a Bonsai Tree
Caroll Hermann states in her doctoral thesis that "There is an ancient Japanese saying that 'tears are dried, pain disappears and heartaches mended when one is pulling weeds or watering a flower'. In ancient Japanese culture, the spiritual rebirth by Nature is contained in the peaceful cultivation of Bonsai" (Hermann 2015). In the near future, Dr. Hermann plans to publish a book about the healing power of cultivating bonsai trees.

Create a Healing Garden
Being exposed to nature can help reduce psychological stress and allow you to heal by promoting relaxation (Mitrione 2008). A garden inspires you to be outside in the fresh air and sunshine, and among serene wildlife, such as butterflies and hummingbirds.

Use your senses to heal your mind and body in your home garden:

- **Touch** various textures of plants, and put your hands in the soil
- **See** an array of colors
- **Listen** to the birds or a backyard waterfall
- **Smell** a variety of plants such as mint, rosemary, and basil
- **Taste** an assortment of teas brewed from garden herbs

Try growing the following in your backyard or greenhouse, or in pots on your porch, balcony, patio, or windowsill:

- *Fruits*—apples, berries, grapes, plums
- *Healing plants*—aloe vera, lavender
- *Herbs*—basil, mint, parsley, rosemary
- *Vegetables*— cucumbers, tomatoes

Engage in Visual Arts
Try your hand at visual arts activities, such as painting, drawing, or pottery, to facilitate the healing process (Stuckey et al. 2010).

Get Adequate Vitamin D

See your physician to get your vitamin D level checked. Vitamin D might help optimize recovery after injury since it is reduced after inflammatory insult (such as knee replacement surgery) and is essential for optimal bone health and muscle function (Bogunovic et al. 2010; Reid et al. 2011; Stratos et al. 2013). An article by Pludowski et al. (2013) states that "adequate vitamin D status seems to be protective against musculoskeletal disorders (muscle weakness, falls, fractures), infectious diseases, autoimmune diseases, cardiovascular disease, type 1 and type 2 diabetes mellitus, several types of cancer, neurocognitive dysfunction and mental illness, and other diseases."

Get Enough Sleep

An article by Patel et al. (2008) indicates that "immune system dysfunction, impaired wound healing, and changes in behavior are all observed in patients who are sleep-deprived."

Get Social Support and Have Hope

A study indicates that "hope and social support are psychological strengths that may be beneficial to an injured athlete's rehabilitation and subjective well-being" (Lu et al. 2013).

Give a Hug

A simple hug can help heal illness, depression, and anxiety. Of course, avoid a hug if a person is contagious and restricted for contact in a medical setting. However, you can resort to laughter and other forms of healing. A study by Matsunaga et al. (2009) suggests that "psychological stress may be reduced and we may feel happiness when we kiss and hug a romantic partner." So go for a single hug, group hug, pet hug, or even hug that tree. Just give a hug. For more information, refer to the Touch Research Institute website at www6.miami.edu/touch-research/.

Go on a Retreat

A study shows spiritual retreats that "included guided imagery, meditation, drumming, journal writing, and nature-based activities" increased hope while reducing depression in individuals with acute coronary syndrome (Warber et al. 2011).

Interact with a Pet

It's no secret that dogs are humans' best friends and we are cats' best friends. Pets can serve as important sources of social support (McConnell et al. 2011), enhance daily living of older individuals (Raina et al. 1999), and help people heal. So, give your hug-gable pet a big squeeze.

Keep a Journal or Diary

The authors of one study (Koschwanez et al. 2013) state that "expressive writing can improve wound healing in older adults and women. Future research is needed to bet-ter understand the underlying cognitive, psychosocial, and biological mechanisms contributing to improved wound healing from these simple, yet effective, writing ex-ercises." Another study by Burton et al. (2004) indicates that "writing about intensely positive experiences was also associated with significantly fewer health center visits for illness."

Keep on the Sunny Side

Wadey et al. (2013) indicates that "as optimism increased, the likelihood of injury oc-currence decreased." Also, optimism can be important for cardiovascular health (Roy et al. 2010).

Let Go of Stress

Studies have shown that controlling acute and chronic stress can have a positive effect on healing (Altemus et al. 2001; Glaser et al. 1999; Kiecolt-Glaser et al. 1995; Stults-Kolehmainen et al. 2014). To relax and reduce stress, simply smile, laugh, whistle, sing, hum, play a fun game, read some comics, or watch a funny movie.

Let Music Mend Your Mind and Body

Music therapy might help reduce pain and anxiety, which can promote speedy heal-ing (Bradt et al. 2013; Nilsson 2008). Refer to the MusicMendsMinds, Inc. website at www.musicmendsminds.org to learn more about the therapeutic benefits of music. Music can help heal the mind and body. Studies have shown that music can decrease pain in an intensive care unit (ICU) setting (Chiasson et al. 2013) and anxiety after heart surgery (Nilsson 2009). A study by Lubetzky et al. (2010) indicates that "expo-sure to Mozart music significantly lowers resting energy expenditure in healthy pre-term infants. We speculate that this effect of music on resting energy expenditure might explain, in part, the improved weight gain that results from this 'Mozart effect.'"

Of course, everyone has his or her own tastes and preferences for music. Consider including the following on your healing playlist:

Bach, Johann Sebastian

- "Brandenburg Concertos"
- "Air on the G String"
- "Goldberg Variations"
- "Suite for Solo Cello No. 1 in G major"

Beethoven, Ludwig van

- "Ode to Joy"
- "Bagatelle No. 25 in A minor (Für Elise)"

Brahms, Johannes

- "Wiegenlied, Op. 49, No. 4 (Lullaby)"

Chopin, Frédéric François

- "Waltz in C-sharp minor, Op. 64, No. 2"
- "Waltz in A minor"
- "Nocturne in E-flat major, Op. 9, No. 2"

Grieg, Edvard

- "Morning Mood, Peer Gynt, Op. 23"

Handel, George Frideric

- "Water Music"

Liszt, Franz
- "Consolations, No. 3"

Massenet, Jules
- "Méditation (Thaïs)"

Mozart, Wolfgang Amadeus

- "Violin Concerto No. 3 in G major, K. 216, II. Adagio"
- "Violin Concerto No. 5 in A major, K. 219, II. Adagio"
- "Piano Concerto No. 21 in C major, K. 467: II. Andante"

Pachelbel, Johann

- "Canon in D major"

Puccini, Giacomo

- "O mio babbino caro"

Rodrigo, Joaquín

- "Concierto de Aranjuez - Adagio"

Saint-Saëns, Camille

- "The Swan–Carnival of the Animals"

Strauss II, Johann

- "The Blue Danube Waltz"

Tchaikovsky, Pyotr Ilyich

- "Piano Concerto No. 1 in B-flat minor, Op. 23"
- "Dance of the Sugar Plum Fairy"

Vivaldi, Antonio

- "The Four Seasons"

According to traditional Chinese medicine (TCM), healing "sounds should actually physically vibrate the targeted organ like an inner-massage" (Voigt 2014). See a TCM practitioner to learn how, in a safe manner, to make your own vocal healing sounds such as these:

- Heart—"Haaaw"
- Kidney—"Chway"
- Liver—"Shooo"
- Lung—"Tzzz"
- Spleen or stomach—"Whooo"
- Triple burner—"Sheee"

You can also create healing sounds with the following tools:

- Baoding balls (Chinese exercise balls for the hands)
- Bells
- Chimes
- Meditation gongs
- Tibetan bowls
- Tingsha (tiny cymbals)

Let Your Mind Heal Your Body

Sometimes our thoughts and approaches to life get in the way of healing and health. By freeing the mind of clutter, the body can focus its energy on healing and well-being. Practice the following (Kross et al. 2014; Rein et al. 1995):

- Nix the negative self-talk
- Resist the urge to judge
- Walk away from arguments
- Lose the stubbornness
- Let go of anger
- Be more tolerant
- Always show respect
- Act more pleasant and kind

Manage Anger

A study by Gouin et al. (2008) indicates that "the impact of anger control on wound healing has clinical relevance. Individuals with low control over the expression of their anger were 4.2 times more likely to take more than four days to heal, compared to those with higher levels of anger control." The authors conclude that "these findings suggest that the ability to regulate the expression of one's anger has a clinically relevant impact on wound healing."

Pray and Meditate
Your personal spiritual beliefs can help you cope with illness (Brown et al. 2009; Crane 2009).

Quit Smoking
A study shows that smokers had less improvement than nonsmokers after lumbar stenosis surgery (Sanden et al. 2011). If this applies to back surgery, it most likely applies to other types of surgery as well as for injuries.

Read or Write a Poem
Let the creation and expression through poetry be your guide for healing (Carroll 2005). Also, refer the National Association for Poetry Therapy website at www.poetrytherapy.org.

See a Manual Therapy Specialist
Manual therapy can help a person heal. This outlines just a few forms and styles of manual therapy used for healing, recovery, and relaxation:

- Acupressure
- BodyTalk, www.bodytalksystem.com
- Craniosacral therapy, www.upledger.com
- Jin Shin (acupressure)
- Joint manipulation
- Joint mobilization
- Manual lymphatic drainage
- Muscle energy techniques
- Myofascial Release, www.myofascialrelease.com
- Reflexology
- Reiki, www.reiki.org
- Rolfing, www.rolf.org
- Shiatsu
- Sports massage

- Swedish massage
- Thai massage
- Trager Approach, www.trager.com
- Trigger point therapy
- Visceral manipulation, www.barralinstitute.com

See a Mental Health Professional
Consider a consultation with a psychologist, counselor, or psychiatrist to heal from within.

See a Physical Rehabilitation Specialist
A specialist such as a physical therapist, occupational therapist, speech therapist, acupuncturist, or chiropractor might provide appropriate healing techniques and strategies, so ask your physician about a possible referral.

See Your Primary Physician
Speak with your physician about medications and other recommended strategies for speeding up the healing process. For example, ask your physician about platelet-rich plasma (PRP) to improve early tendon healing and repair (Lamplot et al. 2014).

Shelf the Alcohol
Alcohol delays the healing of bone and soft tissues such as tendons and muscles (Jung et al. 2011). It's best to wait until you are completely healed after surgery or injury before consuming alcohol even in moderation.

Try Labyrinth Walking
Refer to Labyrinth Walking Program in Part 14.

Try Tai Chi
This gentle martial arts practice might help boost your immune system (Burke et al. 2007).

Try Visualization, Relaxation, and Guided Imagery
These methods before and after surgery promote faster healing and also reduce pain and anxiety (Huddleston 2012). A study by Broadbent et al. (2012) indicates that relaxation and guided imagery prior to surgery "can reduce stress and improve the wound

healing response in surgical patients." A study by Maddison et al. (2012) indicates that guided "imagery intervention improved knee laxity and healing-related neurobiological factors." Also, a study by Cupal et al. (2001) shows that individuals who underwent a guided imagery intervention had "greater knee strength and significantly less reinjury anxiety" after anterior cruciate ligament reconstruction.

Try a Rocking Chair

Rocking chairs are relaxing and comfortable, and might be better than static seating. Rocking causes the feet and ankles to pump blood back to the heart and brain, thus preventing overall stiffness. a rocking chair to help manage pain from trigger points in the gluteus medius, piriformis, gastrocnemius, and soleus muscles (Travell et al. 1992). So, why sit in a standard chair while watching television or reading when you could be rocking away comfortably, especially if the seat is padded? Also, check out hammocks and porch swings for relaxation. We definitely need to reduce sitting time in our culture, but rocking chairs are good alternatives for the times we do sit. Rock on!

Use Healing Recipes

A well-balanced diet *before* and *after* surgery (or injury) is crucial for optimal healing (Kratzing 2011). Micronutrients most important for wound healing include vitamin A, vitamin C, and zinc (Hwang et al. 2012). Vitamin K (good sources are green, leafy vegetables) assists in proper blood clotting, healing of fractures, and protecting against inflammation (Bitensky et al. 1988; Shea 2008). Consult with a dietitian about providing healing recipes for your needs. Refer to the Academy of Nutrition and Dietetics website at www.eatright.org. For information about finding a dietitian specializing in your needs near your home, click the Find an Expert (Registered Dietitian Nutritionist) link.

Heal With Aromatherapy

Aromatherapy is the "therapeutic use of essential oils distilled from plants in baths, as inhalants, or during massage to treat skin conditions, anxiety and stress, headaches, and depression" (Venes 2013). I was introduced to aromatherapy through my parents without even knowing it. When I was in high school, I asked Mom why my pillowcase smelled like lavender and she answered "It helps keep the wolves away so the sheep can sleep." I guess I was a restless sleeper, and she was trying to help. I also remember Dad having me smell fresh-cut lemons to help me feel better when I had the flu or felt nauseated

For safe and effective use of all essential oils, consult with a professional experienced in aromatherapy. The following are examples of oil scents that can have surprising health benefits:

- **Bergamot** might be useful in reducing preoperative anxiety (Ni et al. 2013).
- **Lavender** can be an essential part of the multidisciplinary treatment for pain after a cesarean section (Olapour et al. 2013), might decrease the number of required analgesics following pediatric tonsillectomy (Soltani et al. 2013), and could help alleviate premenstrual emotional symptoms (Matsumoto et al. 2013).
- **Lemon** can be effective in reducing nausea and vomiting during pregnancy (Yavari et al. 2014).
- **Orange** might reduce salivary cortisol and pulse rate due to anxiety during a child's dental treatment (Jafarzadeh et al. 2013).
- **Peppermint** is effective in relieving postoperative nausea or vomiting when used in conjunction with controlled breathing (Sites et al. 2014). Also, local use of peppermint oil may help relieve a tension headache (Kligler et al. 2007).

Other essential oils to consider include basil, cinnamon, clove, cypress, eucalyptus, myrtle, nutmeg, oregano, rosemary, sage, spearmint, and wintergreen.

Heal With Color

An article by Azeemi et al. (2005) indicates that various colors have different healing characteristics. Unfortunately, very few reliable scientific studies show the safety and effectiveness of chromotherapy for treating a variety of medical conditions.

One study by Kim et al. (2013) indicates that "the purpose of human life is to live in peace with mental stability, to design and follow the life goal, to believe that the past and the present are meaningful, to know the value of life why people live, and to promote personal growth through positive relationship with others. Indeed, purpose in life has been linked to the quality of life, including better mental health and happiness. Thus, purpose in life may provide a new treatment target for interventions aimed at enhancing health and well-being." The authors further state that "these results prove that color therapy will improve purpose in life of the patients with post-stroke disability and caregivers."

Further research is needed in this area. However, for the purpose of this book, consider using color generically and according to your personal preferences for enhancing your mood. For example, red, yellow, and orange can be thought of for stimulation and excitement, and blue and violet for relaxation. Pink, on the other hand, is thought to reduce aggression (Schauss 1979, 1985).

Observe some art and photographs to help soothe your mind and body. A study shows that nurses can use photographic imagery, such as a lake sunset, rocky river, or an autumn waterfall, as a restorative intervention in a hospital setting (Hanson et al. 2013).

Heal With Honey
Products of the honeybee include bee venom, honey, pollen, royal jelly, propolis, and beeswax. According to the American Apitherapy Society, apitherapy (from the Latin *apis*, which means "bee") is the medicinal use of products made by honeybees.

Honey can benefit wound healing (Weissenstein et al. 2014), reduce post tonsillectomy pain (Mohebbi et al. 2014), and has antioxidant and anti-inflammatory properties (Alvarez-Suarez et al. 2013) when used under the supervision of a medical practitioner.

A study by Paul et al. (2007) also indicates that buckwheat "honey may be a preferable treatment for the cough and sleep difficulty associated with childhood upper respiratory tract infection." Another study by Watanabe et al. (2014) indicates that "honey, in general, and particularly manuka honey, has potent inhibitory activity against the influenza virus."

Check with your healthcare provider before using honey for any medical conditions since honey can negatively interact with certain medications, increase blood sugar, and cause allergic reactions in some people who are prone.

Heal With Water
Many cultures, such as the traditional Romans and Greeks, have long used the healing effects of water for recovery and recuperation. Consider the following forms of healing in water:

- Ai Chi
- Aquatic therapy
- Bad Ragaz Ring Method, www.badragazringmethod.org/en
- Balneotherapy
- Halliwick Aquatic Therapy, http://halliwick.org

- Hot tubs and spas (such as a Jacuzzi)
- Hydrotherapy
- Thalassotherapy
- Watsu, www.watsu.com
- Whirlpool bath

Other forms of healing waters can be found in these basic activities:

- Fishing
- Listening to waterfalls (outdoors or in the home)
- Sailing
- Scuba diving
- Swimming

Wear Compression Garments
Ask your healthcare provider about compression garments and clothing to help you with healing and recovery (Armstrong et al. 2015; Goto et al. 2014; Kraemer et al. 2010).

Did You Know?

- "Regeneration in most tissues refers to the replacement of tissue by cell division; neural regeneration refers to the growth of damaged axons. Axotomized peripheral nervous system axons can regenerate at the rate of approximately 1 mm/day" (Aminoff et al. 2013; Castro et al. 2002; Sunderland 1991).
- Majority of nonoperative extremity fractures heal in 4 to 8 weeks (McKinnis 2014).
- A fully mature fibrous scar requires 12 to 18 months [for healing] and is about 20% to 30% weaker than normal skin" (Goodman et al. 2015).
- It is safe to adopt a 'wait-and-watch' policy for cases of massive disc herniation if there is any early sign of clinical improvement. Initial follow-up at an average of 23.2 months revealed that 83% had a complete and sustained recovery at the initial follow-up. A massive disc herniation can pursue a favorable clinical course. If early progress is shown, the long-term prognosis is very good and even massive disc herniation's can be treated conservatively (Benson et al. 2010).

- "Joint effusion increases intraarticular pressure and afferent activity, which contributes to muscle inhibition. In fact, even small increases in fluid in a joint (as little as 10 mL) can produce a 50% to 60% decrease in maximal voluntary contractions of the quadriceps" (Andrews et al. 2012, p. 43). In other words, knee swelling may cause your knee to give out while walking.

Final Words

Some additional factors that influence healing include the following: age; coexisting conditions such as diabetes, presence of infection, types of tissue involved (muscle, tendon, ligament, bone, or skin), types of trauma, medications, and hormones.

Also, keep in mind the wise words of Norman Cousins, an American political journalist: "In the healing equation, therefore, the physician brings the best that medical science has to offer, and the patient brings the best that millions of years of evolution have to offer" (Carlson et al. 1989).

Additional Resources

- All Things Healing, www.allthingshealing.com
- American Art Therapy Association, www.arttherapy.org
- American Music Therapy Association, www.musictherapy.org
- Animal Planet, www.animalplanet.com
- Healing Guide Retreats and Escapes, www.healingguide.org
- Healing Lifestyles & Spas, www.healinglifestyles.com
- Music Heals, www.music-heals.com
- Spine Surgery Recovery, www.spine-surgery-recovery.com
- Vitamin D Council, www.vitamindcouncil.org
- Wound Healing Society, http://woundheal.org

References

Al-Sharman A, and Siengsukon CF. (2013). Sleep enhances learning of a functional motor task in young adults. *Physical Therapy* 93 (12): 1625–1635.

Altemus M, Rao B, Dhabhar FS, et al. (2001). Stress-induced changes in skin barrier function in healthy women. *Journal of Investigative Dermatology* 117 (2): 309–317.

Aminoff MJ, Boller F, and Swaab DF. (Eds.). (2013). *Peripheral Nerve Disorders* (Volume 115, 3rd Series). New York, NY: Elsevier.

Andrews JR, Harrelson GL, Wilk KE. (2012). *Physical Rehabilitation of the Injured Athlete*, 4th ed. Philadelphia, PA: Elsevier Saunders.

Armstrong SA, Till ES, Maloney SR, et al. (2015). Compression socks and functional recovery following marathon running: A randomized controlled trial. *Journal of Strength and Conditioning Research* 29 (2): 528–533.

Azeemi ST, and Raza SM. (2005). A critical analysis of chromotherapy and its scientific evolution. *Evidence-based Complementary and Alternative* 2 (4): 481–488.

Beauchemin KM, and Hays P. (1996). Sunny hospital rooms expedite recovery from severe and refractory depressions. *Journal of Affective Disorders* 40 (1–2): 49–51.

Beauchemin KM, and Hays P. (1998). Dying in the dark: Sunshine, gender and outcomes in myocardial infarction. *Journal of the Royal Society of Medicine* 91 (7): 352–354.

Benson RT, Tavares SP, Robertson SC, et al. (2010). Conservatively treated massive prolapsed discs: A 7-year follow-up. *Ann R Coll Surg Engl* 92 (2): 147-153.

Bitensky L, Hart JP, Catterall A, et al. (1988). Circulating vitamin K levels in patients with fractures. *Journal of Bone and Joint Surgery. British Volume* 70 (4): 663–664.

Bogunovic L, Kim AD, Beamer BS, et al. (2010). Hypovitaminosis D in patients scheduled to undergo orthopaedic surgery: A single-center analysis. *Journal of Bone and Joint Surgery. American Volume* 92 (13): 2300–2304.

Bradt J, Dileo C, and Shim M. (2013). Music interventions for preoperative anxiety. *Cochrane Database of Systematic Reviews* 6, Cd006908.

Broadbent E, Kahokehr A, Booth RJ, et al. (2012). A brief relaxation intervention reduces stress and improves surgical wound healing response: A randomised trial. *Brain, Behavior and Immunity* 26 (2): 212–217.

Brown RP, and Gerbarg PL. (2009). Yoga breathing, meditation, and longevity. *Annals of the New York Academy of Sciences* 1172: 54–62.

Burke DT, Al-Adawi S, Lee YT, et al. (2007). Martial arts as sport and therapy. *Journal of Sports Medicine and Physical Fitness* 47 (1): 96–102.

Burton CM, and King LA. (2004). The health benefits of writing about intensely positive experiences. *Journal of Research in Personality* 38 (2): 150–163.

Carlson R, and Shield B. (1989). *Healers on Healing*. Los Angeles, CA: Jeremy P. Tarcher, Inc.

Carroll R. (2005). Finding the words to say it: The healing power of poetry. *Evidence-Based Complementary and Alternative Medicine* 2 (2): 161–172.

Castro AJ, Merchut MP, Neafsey EJ, et al. (2002). *Neuroscience: An Outline Approach.* St. Louis, MO: Mosby.

Chiasson AM, Linda Baldwin A, McLaughlin C, et al. (2013). The effect of live spontaneous harp music on patients in the intensive care unit. *Evidence-based and Complementary and Alternative Medicine* 2013: 428731.

Crane JN. (2009). Religion and cancer: Examining the possible connections. *Journal of Psychosocial Oncology* 27 (4): 469–486.

Cupal DD, and Brewer BW. (2001). Effects of relaxation and guided imagery on knee strength, reinjury anxiety, and pain following anterior cruciate ligament reconstruction. *Rehabilitation Psychology* 46 (1): 28–43.

dos Santos Alves VL, Alves da Silva RJ, and Avanzi O. (2014). Effect of a preoperative protocol of aerobic physical therapy on the quality of life of patients with adolescent idiopathic scoliosis: A randomized clinical study. *American Journal of Orthopedics (Belle Mead NJ)* 43 (6): E112–116.

Glaser R, Kiecolt-Glaser JK, Marucha PT, et al. (1999). Stress-related changes in proinflammatory cytokine production in wounds. *Archives of General Psychiatry* 56 (5): 450–456.

Goodman CC, Fuller KS. (2015). *Pathology: Implications for the Physical Therapist*, 4th ed. St. Louis, MO: Saunders Elsevier.

Goto K, and Morishima T. (2014). Compression garment promotes muscular strength recovery after resistance exercise. *Medicine and Science in Sports and Exercise* 46 (12): 2265–2270.

Gouin JP, Kiecolt-Glaser JK, Malarkey WB, et al. (2008). The influence of anger expression on wound healing. *Brain Behavior and Immunity* 22 (5): 699–708.

Gyulai F, Raba K, Baranyai I, et al. (2015). BEMER therapy combined with physiotherapy in patients with musculoskeletal diseases: A randomised, controlled double blind follow-up pilot study. *Evidence-Based Complementary and Alternative Medicine* 245742.

Hanson H, Schroeter K, Hanson A, et al. (2013). Preferences for photographic art among hospitalized patients with cancer. *Oncology Nursing Forum* 40 (4): E337–345.

Hermann C. (2015). *Integral ecospychological investigation of bonsai principles, meaning and healing.* (Unpublished doctoral thesis). University of Zululand, South Africa.

Hoogeboom TJ, Dronkers JJ, Hulzebos EH, et al. (2014). Merits of exercise therapy before and after major surgery. *Current Opinion in Anaesthesiology* 27 (2): 161–166.

Huddleston P. (2012). *Prepare for Surgery, Heal Faster: A Guide of Mind-Body Techniques*, 4th ed. Cambridge, MA: Angel River Press.

Humphrey R, and Malone D. (2015). Effectiveness of preoperative physical therapy for elective cardiac surgery. *Physical Therapy* 95 (2): 160–166.

Hwang C, Ross V, and Mahadevan U. (2012). Micronutrient deficiencies in inflammatory bowel disease: From A to zinc. *Inflammatory Bowel Diseases* 18 (10): 1961–1981.

Jafarzadeh M, Arman S, and Pour FF. (2013). Effect of aromatherapy with orange essential oil on salivary cortisol and pulse rate in children during dental treatment: A randomized controlled clinical trial. *Advanced Biomedical Research* 2: 10.

Jung MK, Callaci JJ, Lauing KL, et al. (2011). Alcohol exposure and mechanisms of tissue injury and repair. *Alcoholism, Clinical and Experimental Research* 35 (3): 392–399.

Kiecolt-Glaser K, Marucha PT, Malarkey WB, et al. (1995). Slowing of wound healing by psychological stress. *Lancet* 346 (8984): 1194–1196.

Kim MK, and Kang SD. (2013). Effects of art therapy using color on purpose in life in patients with stroke and their caregivers. *Yonsei Medical Journal* 54 (1): 15–20.

Kligler B, and Chaudhary S. (2007). Peppermint oil. *American Family Physician* 75 (7): 1027–1030.

Koschwanez HE, Kerse N, Darragh M, et al. (2013). Expressive writing and wound healing in older adults: a randomized controlled trial. *Psychosomatic Medicine* 75 (6): 581–590.

Kraemer WJ, Flanagan SD, Comstock BA, et al. (2010). Effects of a whole body compression garment on markers of recovery after a heavy resistance workout in men and women. *Journal of Strength and Conditioning Research.* 24 (3): 804–814.

Kratzing C. (2011). Preoperative nutrition and carbohydrate loading. *Proceedings of the Nutrition Society* 70 (3): 311–315.

Kross E, Bruehlman-Senecal E, Park J., et al. (2014). Self-talk as a regulatory mechanism: How you do it matters. *Journal of Personality and Social Psychology* 106 (2): 304–324.

Lamplot JD, Angeline M, Angeles J, et al. (2014). Distinct effects of platelet-rich plasma and BMP13 on rotator cuff tendon injury healing in a rat model. *American Journal of Sports Medicine* 42 (12): 2877–2887.

Lu FJH, and Hsu Y. (2013). Injured athletes' rehabilitation beliefs and subjective well-being: The contribution of hope and social support. *Journal of Athletic Training* 48 (1): 92–98.

Lubetzky R, Mimouni FB, Dollberg S, et al. (2010). Effect of music by Mozart on energy expenditure in growing preterm infants. *Pediatrics.* 125 (1): e24–28.

Maddison R, Prapavessis H, Clatworthy M, et al. (2012). Guided imagery to improve functional outcomes post-anterior cruciate ligament repair: Randomized-controlled pilot trial. *Scandinavian Journal of Medicine & Science in Sports* 22 (6): 816–821.

Matsunaga M, Sato S, Isowa T, et al. (2009). Profiling of serum proteins influenced by warm partner contact in healthy couples. *Neuro Endocrinology Letters* 30 (2): 227–236.

Matsumoto T, Asakura H, and Hayashi T. (2013). Does lavender aromatherapy alleviate premenstrual emotional symptoms? A randomized crossover trial. *BioPsychoSocial Medicine* 7: 12.

McConnell AR, Brown CM, Shoda TM, et al. (2011). Friends with benefits: On the positive consequences of pet ownership. *Journal of Personality and Social Psychology* 101 (6): 1239–1252.

McCulloch JM, and Kloth LC. (2010). *Wound Healing: Evidence-Based Management*, 4th ed. Philadelphia, PA: FA Davis.

McKinnis L. (2014). *Fundamental of Musculoskeletal Imaging, 4th ed.* Philadelphia, PA: FA Davis Company.

Mitrione S. (2008). Therapeutic responses to natural environments: Using gardens to improve health care. *Minnesota Medicine* 91 (3): 31–34.

Ni CH, Hou WH, Kao CC, et al. (2013). The anxiolytic effect of aromatherapy on patients awaiting ambulatory surgery: A randomized controlled trial. *Evidence-based Complementary and Alternative Medicine* 927419.

Nilsson U. (2008). The anxiety- and pain-reducing effects of music interventions: A systematic review. *Association of Operating Room Nurses Journal* 87 (4): 780–807.

Nilsson U. (2009). Soothing music can increase oxytocin levels during bed rest after open-heart surgery: A randomised control trial. *Journal of Clinical Nursing* 18 (15): 2153–2161.

Olapour A, Behaeen K, Akhondzadeh R, et al. (2013). The effect of inhalation of aromatherapy blend containing lavender essential oil on cesarean postoperative pain. *Anesthesiology and Pain Medicine* 3 (1): 203–207.

Patel M, Chipman J, Carlin BW, et al. (2008). Sleep in the intensive care unit setting. *Critical Care Nursing Quarterly* 31 (4): 309–318.

Paul IM, Beiler J, McMonagle A, et al. (2007). Effect of honey, dextromethorphan, and no treatment on nocturnal cough and sleep quality for coughing children and their parents. *Archives of Pediatric & Adolescent Medicine* 161 (12): 1140–1146.

Piatkowski J, Kern S, and Ziemssen T. (2009). Effect of BEMER magnetic field therapy on the level of fatigue in patients with multiple sclerosis: A randomized, double-blind controlled trial. *Journal of Alternative and Complementary Medicine* 15 (5): 507–511.

Pludowski P, Holick MF, Pilz S, et al. (2013). Vitamin D effects on musculoskeletal health, immunity, autoimmunity, cardiovascular disease, cancer, fertility, pregnancy, dementia and mortality-A review of recent evidence. *Autoimmunity Reviews* 12 (10): 976–989.

Raina P, Waltner-Toews D, Bonnett B, et al. (1999). Influence of companion animals on the physical and psychological health of older people: An analysis of a one-year longitudinal study. *Journal of the American Geriatrics Society* 47 (3): 323–329.

Reid D, Toole BJ, Knox S, et al. (2011). The relation between acute changes in the systemic inflammatory response and plasma 25-hydroxyvitamin D concentrations after elective knee arthroplasty. *American Journal of Clinical Nutrition* 93 (5): 1006–1011.

Rein G, Atkinson M, and McCraty R. (1995). The physiological and psychological effects of compassion and anger. *Journal of Advancement in Medicine* 8 (2): 87–105.

Roy B, Diez-Roux AV, Seeman T, et al. (2010). Association of optimism and pessimism with inflammation and hemostasis in the Multi-Ethnic Study of Atherosclerosis (MESA). *Psychosomatic Medicine* 72 (2): 134–140.

Sandén B, Försth P, and Michaëlsson K. (2011). Smokers show less improvement than non-smokers 2 years after surgery for lumbar spinal stenosis: A study of 4555 patients from the Swedish spine register. *Spine (Philadelphia, Pa. 1976)* 36 (13): 1059–1064.

Schauss AG. (1979). Tranquilizing effect of color reduces aggressive behavior and potential violence. *Orthomolecular Psychiatry* 8 (4): 218–221.

Schauss AG. (1985). The physiological effect of color on the suppression of human aggression: Research on Baker-Miller pink. *International Journal for Biosocial Research* 7 (2): 55–64.

Shea MK, Booth SL, Massaro JM, et al. (2008). Vitamin K and vitamin D status: Associations with inflammatory markers in the Framingham Offspring Study. *American Journal of Epidemiology* 167 (3): 313–320.

Siengsukon CF, and Boyd LA. (2009). Does sleep promote motor learning? Implications for physical rehabilitation. *Physical Therapy* 89 (4): 370–383.

Sites DS, Johnson NT, Miller JA, et al. (2014). Controlled breathing with or without peppermint aromatherapy for postoperative nausea and/or vomiting symptom relief: A randomized controlled trial. *Journal of Perianesthesia Nursing* 29 (1): 12–19.

Soltani R, Soheilipour S, Hajhashemi V, et al. (2013). Evaluation of the effect of aromatherapy with lavender essential oil on post-tonsillectomy pain in pediatric patients: A randomized controlled trial. *International Journal of Pediatric Otorhinolaryngology* 77 (9): 1579–1581.

Stratos I, Li Z, Herlyn P, Rotter R, et al. (2013). Vitamin D increases cellular turnover and functionally restores the skeletal muscle after crush injury in rats. *American Journal Pathology* 182 (3): 895–904.

Stuckey HL, and Nobel J. (2010). The connection between art, healing, and public health: A review of current literature. *American Journal of Public Health* 100 (2): 254–263.

Stults-Kolehmainen MA, Bartholomew JB, and Sinha R. (2014). Chronic psychological stress impairs recovery of muscular function and somatic sensations over a 96-hour period. *Journal of Strength and Conditioning Research* 28 (7): 2007–2017.

Sunderland S. (1991). *Nerve Injuries and Their Repair: A Critical Appraisal.* London, England: WB Saunders Company.

Travell JG, and Simons DG. (1992). *Travell & Simons' Myofascial Pain and Dysfunction: The Trigger Point Manual.* (Volume 2)—The Lower Extremities. Baltimore MD: Williams & Wilkins.

Vaajoki A, Pietilä AM, Kankkunen P, et al. (2012). Effects of listening to music on pain intensity and pain distress after surgery: An intervention. *Journal of Clinical Nursing* 21 (5–6): 708–17.

Venes D. (Ed.). (2013). *Taber's Cyclopedic Medical Dictionary,* 22nd ed. Philadelphia, PA: FA Davis.

Wadey R, Evans L, Hanton S, et al. (2013). Effect of dispositional optimism before and after injury. *Medicine and Science in Sports and Exercise* 45 (2): 387–394.

Warber SL, Ingerman S, Moura VL, et al. (2011). Healing the heart: A randomized pilot study of a spiritual retreat for depression in acute coronary syndrome patients. *Explore (NY)* 7 (4): 222–233.

Watanabe K, Rahmasari R, Matsunaga A, et al. (2014). Anti-influenza viral effects of honey in vitro: Potent high activity of manuka honey. *Archives of Medical Research* 45 (5): 359–365.

Weissenstein A, Luchter E, and Bittmann S. (2014). Medical honey and its role in paediatric patients. *British Journal of Nursing* 23 (6): S30, s32–34.

Yavari Kia P, Safajou F, Shahnazi M, et al. (2014). The effect of lemon inhalation aromatherapy on nausea and vomiting of pregnancy: A double-blinded, randomized, controlled clinical trial. *Iranian Red Crescent Medical Journal* 16 (3): e14360.

Xie L, Kang H, Xu Q, et al. (2013). Sleep drives metabolite clearance from the adult brain. *Science* 342

PART 2
Getting Enough Sleep

Getting enough sleep every night is essential for good health. The earlier stages of sleep are necessary for physical repair (such as muscle repair and organ cleansing) while the later stages of sleep are important for psychological repair (such as laying down memory in the brain and working through anxiety) (University of Michigan Health System 2003).

Chronic sleep problems can increase your risk of heart attack, stroke, high blood pressure, diabetes, depression, and other medical problems. A person could lose sleep because he or she is in pain, is taking certain medications, has uncontrolled stress and worry, is undergoing hormonal changes (such as menopause), has just had surgery, or has poor sleeping habits. Quality of sleep is considered good when a person can fall asleep relatively quickly (within five to 15 minutes), wake up easily, stay asleep almost continuously, and sleep long enough to feel refreshed the next day (Akerstedt et al. 1997).

The following list sheds light on potential problems in those who don't get enough sleep (Ancoli-Israel et al. 2005; Cohen et al. 2009; Kundermann et al. 2004; Stone et al. 2008; UCLA Conference 2009, 2010; Walker 2009):

- Daytime fatigue, low energy, physical and mental tiredness, and weariness
- Mood disturbances
- Impaired cognitive functioning
- Impaired memory and concentration
- Difficulty sustaining attention with tasks
- Slowed response times (good reaction times are critical for safe driving, safety at work, and preventing falls)

- Increased incidence of colds and viruses, and a weakened immune system
- Increased pain perception
- Increased risk of falls
- Decreased job performance
- Reduced quality of life and inability to enjoy social relationships
- Shorter life span
- A possible role in the current obesity epidemic
- Decreased safety on the road, leading to car crashes

Research says...

- Mindfulness meditation improves sleep quality in older adults (Black et al. 2015).
- A study by Grigsby-Toussaint et al. (2015) indicates that in order to obtain enough quality sleep, get outside to a park or trail or take a walk around a local high school or college campus.
- A study by Prather et al. (2015) found that sleeping 7 or more hours may help reduce susceptibility to the common cold.
- A study by Cai et al. (2014) indicates that regular moderate- to high-intensity step aerobics training "can improve sleep quality and increase the melatonin levels in sleep-impaired postmenopausal women."
- Elite athletes should consider the fact that early-morning training programs reduce sleep duration and increase pre-training fatigue levels (Sargent et al. 2014).
- A study by Al-Sharman et al. (2013) indicates that "sleep facilitates learning clinically relevant functional motor tasks."
- Waste removal may be one of the fundamental reasons for sleep (Xie et al. 2013).
- A study by Siengsukon et al. (2009) indicates that despite certain unanswered questions in sleep research, "therapists should consider encouraging sleep following therapy sessions as well as promoting healthy sleep in their patients with chronic stroke to promote offline motor learning of the skills practiced during rehabilitation."

25 Rules for Choosing Snoozing
Here's a list of rules to follow to help you improve sleep habits and nighttime rituals for a good night's sleep (Avidan 2010; Bloom et al. 2009; Kryger et al. 2005; UCLA Conference 2009, 2010; University of Michigan Health System 2003):

RULE 1: GET ENOUGH SLEEP EVERY NIGHT

Most adults need around seven to eight hours of sleep every night, while adolescents might need up to nine or 10 hours (University of Michigan Health System 2003).

RULE 2: ESTABLISH BEDTIME HABITS

Have regular bedtime and waking hours by going to bed when sleepy, at a relatively consistent time, and getting up at the same time each day to synchronize your body clock.

RULE 3: CREATE A COMFY ROOM

Make sure your room is dark, quiet, and cool but comfortable. In most cases, room temperatures below 54 degrees Fahrenheit and higher than 75 degrees Fahrenheit will disrupt sleep (National Sleep Foundation 2013). Also, keep the room well ventilated.

RULE 4: SLEEP IN A COMFY BED

Make sure your bed, blankets, sheets, and pillows feel comfortable to you. Also, be sure you have a mattress that meets your needs.

RULE 5: HAVE NO TIME CONSTRAINTS

Turn your alarm clock so it does not face your bed, since time pressure of clock-watching might contribute to poor sleep (Ancoli-Israel 1996). This also keeps the clock light from disturbing you.

RULE 6: EMBRACE MINDLESSNESS BEFORE BED

Allow at least one hour to unwind before bedtime (Kryger et al. 2005) by avoiding, during that time, stimulating activities such as watching a movie, reading an intense book, emotional discussions, or playing competitive games like chess.

RULE 7: TONE DOWN THE MUSIC

Avoid intense or fast-paced music close to bedtime since it acts as a stimulant. However, do listen to music that is soothing and relaxing. Go to bed with a relaxed mind.

RULE 8: STAY OFF THE INTERNET

A study shows that computer use between 7:00 p.m. and midnight increases risk of poor sleep among young adults. Mesquita et al. (2010) state that "the strength, variation, and timing of light projected onto the retina by these devices [computers] disrupt the normal release of melatonin in the body (the hormone that controls sleep), resulting in changes in quality of sleep." Another study by Lemola et al. (2015) states that "excessive electronic media [smartphone] use at night is a risk factor for both adolescents' [ages 12–17 years old] sleep disturbance and depression."

RULE 9: TURN OFF THE RADIO AND TELEVISION BEFORE FALLING ASLEEP
Keeping the radio and television turned on to help a person fall asleep can ultimately disrupt sleep (Gooneratne et al. 2011). The external stimuli of sound and light does not allow for relaxation. A quiet, dark room is best for falling asleep—and staying asleep.

RULE 10: DO WHAT'S RELAXING, NOT TAXING
Engage in relaxing activities 20 to 30 minutes before sleep (Attarian 2010). Try gentle yoga, tai chi, qigong, relaxation techniques, or mindfulness training (see Part 13). Teach your mind and body that your bed is for relaxation, not frustration.

RULE 11: EXERCISE REGULARLY
A study by Reid et al. (2010) indicates that engaging in moderate aerobic physical activity generally improves "sleep quality, mood, and quality of life in older adults with chronic insomnia." Another study indicates that vigorous late-night exercise on a stationary bicycle did not disturb sleep in young and fit individuals without sleep disorders (Myllymäki et al. 2011). However, sleep researchers typically agree that intense exercise close to bedtime acts as a stimulant and might prevent you from getting a good night's sleep. Get regular exercise in the afternoon or early evening, but avoid it close to bedtime (Kryger et al. 2005).

RULE 12: ABSORB BRIGHT MORNING LIGHT
Early bright light exposure is very helpful in synchronizing your body clock and helping to wake you in the morning—the best source is sunlight (Ancoli-Israel et al. 2005). If you can't get outdoors early in the morning, have breakfast near a window or on a balcony, porch, or patio. The timing of bright light exposure might be adjusted to late afternoon or evening by a sleep medicine physician if a patient has certain difficulties, such as falling asleep too early, working late shifts, or is a frequent jet traveler (Zee et al. 2010).

RULE 13: MAKE YOUR BED A SLEEP-ONLY ZONE
Do not watch television, read, write, eat, talk on the telephone, use your laptop, or play board games on your bed.

RULE 14: USE CAUTION WITH NAPS

Consider avoiding daytime naps if you have difficulty with nighttime sleep. If you are unsure about napping during the day, discuss the benefits of napping with your physician. However, avoid naps close to bedtime. If you do take a nap, try to keep it around 10 to 30 minutes in the afternoon (Brooks et al. 2006; Milner et al. 2009).

RULE 15: PASS UP CERTAIN FOODS

Avoid foods such as aged cheeses, spicy foods, smoked meats, and ginseng tea near bedtime since they might keep you awake. On the other hand, a study shows that eating two kiwifruits one hour before bedtime might help individuals with sleep disturbances fall asleep (Lin et al. 2011).

RULE 16: CUT OUT CAFFEINE

Avoid caffeinated foods and beverages (coffee, tea, chocolate, sodas, or colas) close to bedtime since caffeine is a stimulant and disturbs sleep (Attarian 2010). The effects of caffeine can remain in the body for three to five hours (Ancoli-Israel 1996).

RULE 17: BID BYE-BYE TO TOBACCO

Avoid smoking and other tobacco products within two hours of bedtime since nicotine is a stimulant that disturbs sleep. Better yet, give up smoking altogether for myriad health benefits.

RULE 18: NIX THE NIGHTCAP

Consuming alcohol near bedtime fragments and disrupts sleep (Kryger et al. 2005; Van Reen et al. 2011). Also, a study indicates that stopping alcohol consumption at bedtime can improve sleep conditions (Morita et al. 2012). Another study by Jefferson et al. (2005) indicates that "insomniacs do engage in specific poor sleep hygiene practices, such as smoking and drinking alcohol just before bedtime."

RULE 19: EAT DINNER IN THE EARLY EVENING

Avoid late, heavy meals within three hours of bedtime. The key is not to go to bed hungry or too full. A heavy meal can cause indigestion or heartburn and, thus, keep you awake.

RULE 20: GO EASY ON THE FLUIDS

Avoid excess consumption of fluids within two hours of bedtime to prevent frequent bathroom trips at night (Attarian 2010).

RULE 21: TAKE MEDS LIKE CLOCKWORK

Since many prescription and over-the-counter medicines can affect sleep, take your medications according to your physician's instructions. Don't vary your medication times unless directed by your physician or pharmacist.

RULE 22: TAKE A BEDTIME BATHROOM BREAK

Empty your bladder (and bowels, if necessary) before going to sleep to prevent bathroom trips that can interfere with sleep.

RULE 23: CAN'T SLEEP? GET UP

Getting to sleep should be effortless and not forced. If you don't fall asleep within 20 minutes, get out of bed and do something relaxing. Counting sheep to sleep is unlikely to help. Try gentle stretching, five to 10 minutes of yoga, mindfulness meditation, or listening to soothing music. You can also try imagery distraction (Harvey et al. 2002), which entails imagining a situation you find interesting and engaging (such as relaxing at the beach with your feet in warm sand, sitting in a cozy chair on top of a mountain overlooking a distant lake, or swinging in a hammock between two palm trees and listening to the gentle waves breaking on the shore).

RULE 24: BE CAREFUL WITH SHARING

Sharing your bed with your children or pets can disturb your (and their) sleep.

RULE 25: SAY NO TO SLEEPING PILLS

Always consult with your physician before using over-the-counter sleeping pills.

Sample Sleep Preparation Routine

In practical terms, 16 hours of reality is enough. It's time for pleasant dreams and sleepy time. The body needs patterns and cycles to thrive. The following is a simple sleep routine you can use to help get a good night's sleep. Please feel free to change the order and elements according to your needs:

- Power down all your electronic devices.
- Take care of toilet needs.
- Wash your hands and face, and brush and floss teeth.

- Groom and talk to your pet. He has been waiting all day to hear about your adventures.
- Smell a little scent of lavender oil to relax.
- Gently massage your neck, back, and foot for one minute.
- Turn off all the lights.
- Feel your back on your cozy bed and the warm blankets over you.
- Take a moment of silence through prayer or personal reflection to be grateful for another day.
- Sleep tight.

Acupressure Routine for Relaxation

See an acupuncturist for detailed instructions. Try the following points for three minutes each to help you relax (Harris et al. 2005):

- Anmian point—lightly tap behind the ear (posterior to the mastoid process).
- Yin Tang point—massage the area between your eyebrows.
- Ht 7 point—massage with your thumb on the palm and little finger side where your wrist forms a crease with your hand.
- Liv 3 point—massage the middle top portion of your foot between the first and second toes.
- Sp 6 point—massage the inside of your lower leg about four fingers above your inner ankle bone, behind the shin bone.

For further information about healthy sleep habits, talk to your family physician and obtain information from a local sleep disorders clinic. If you have severe difficulty with sleeping, your physician might recommend treatment using biofeedback therapy or cognitive behavioral therapy, or refer you to a sleep lab to obtain more information.

Additional Resources

- American Academy of Sleep Medicine, www.aasmnet.org
- American Sleep Association, www.sleepassociation.org
- National Sleep Foundation, www.sleepfoundation.org

- Sleep to Live Institute, http://sleeptoliveinstitute.com
- Sleepnet.com, www.sleepnet.com
- The Better Sleep Council, www.bettersleep.org
- Refer to the National Institutes of Health, www.nih.gov (search for Sleepless in America).

References

Akerstedt T, Hume K, Minors D, et al. (1997). Good sleep—its timing and physiological sleep characteristics. *Journal of Sleep Research* 6 (4): 221–229.

Al-Sharman A, and Siengsukon CF. (2013). Sleep enhances learning of a functional motor task in young adults. *Physical Therapy* 93 (12): 1625–1635.

Ancoli-Israel S. (1996). *All I Want Is a Good Night's Sleep*. St. Louis, MO: Mosby-Yearbook.

Ancoli-Israel S, and Cooke JR. (2005). Prevalence and comorbidity of insomnia and effect on functioning in elderly populations. *Journal of the American Geriatrics Society* 53 (Supplement 7): S264–71.

Attarian HP. (2010). *Sleep Disorders in Women: A Guide to Practical Management*. Totowa, New Jersey: Humana Press.

Avidan AY. (2010). Sleep medicine rules of sleep hygiene. Personal e-mail communication with author, September 25, 2010.

Black DS, O'Reilly GA, Olmstead R, et al. (2015). Mindfulness meditation and improvement in sleep quality and daytime impairment among older adults with sleep disturbances: A randomized clinical trial. *JAMA Internal Medicine* 175 (4): 494–501.

Bloom HG, Ahmed I, Alessi CA, et al. (2009). Evidence-based recommendations for the assessment and management of sleep disorders in older persons. *Journal of the American Geriatrics Society* 57 (5): 761–789.

Brooks A, and Lack L. (2006). A brief afternoon nap following nocturnal sleep restriction: Which nap duration is most recuperative? *Sleep* 29 (6): 831–840.

Cai ZY, Wen-Chyuan Chen K, and Wen HJ. (2014). Effects of a group-based step aerobics training on sleep quality and melatonin levels in sleep-impaired postmenopausal women. *Journal of Strength and Conditioning Research* 28 (9): 2597–2603.

Cohen S, Doyle WJ, Alper CM, et al. (2009). Sleep habits and susceptibility to the common cold. *Archives of Internal Medicine* 169 (1): 62–67.

Epstein L, and Mardon S. (2007). *Harvard Medical School Guide to a Good Night's Sleep*. New York, NY: McGraw-Hill.

Gooneratne NS, Tavaria A, Patel N, et al. (2011). Perceived effectiveness of diverse sleep treatments in older adults. *Journal of the American Geriatrics Society* 59 (2): 297–303.

Grigsby-Toussaint DS, Turi KN, Krupa M, et al. (2015). Sleep insufficiency and the natural environment: Results from the US Behavioral Risk Factor Surveillance System survey. *Preventive Medicine* 78: 78–84.

Harris RE, Jeter J, Chan P, et al. (2005). Using acupressure to modify alertness in the classroom: A single-blinded, randomized, cross-over trial. *Journal of Alternative and Complementary Medicine* 11 (4): 673–679.

Harvey AG, and Payne S. (2002). The management of unwanted pre-sleep thoughts in insomnia: Distraction with imagery versus general distraction. *Behaviour Research and Therapy* 40 (3): 267–277.

Hereford JM. (2014). *Sleep and Rehabilitation: A Guide for Health Professionals.* Thorofare, NJ: SLACK.

Jefferson CD, Drake CL, Scofield HM, et al. (2005). Sleep hygiene practices in a population-based sample of insomniacs. *Sleep* 28 (5): 611–615.

Kryger MH, Roth T, and Dement WC. (2005). *Principles and Practice of Sleep Medicine,* 4th ed. Philadelphia, PA: Elsevier Saunders.

Kundermann B, Krieg JC, Schreiber W, et al. (2004). The effect of sleep deprivation on pain. *Pain Research & Management* 9 (1): 25–32.

Kushida CA (Ed.). (2008). *Handbook of Sleep Disorders,* 2nd ed. Boca Raton, FL: CRC Press.

Lemola S, Perkinson-Gloor N, Brand S, et al. (2015). Adolescents' electronic media use at night, sleep disturbance, and depressive symptoms in the smartphone age. *Journal of Youth and Adolescence* 44 (2): 405–418.

Lin HH, Tsai PS, Fang SC, et al. (2011). Effect of kiwifruit consumption on sleep quality in adults with sleep problems. *Asia Pacific Journal of Clinical Nutrition.* 20 (2): 169–174.

Mednick SC, and Ehrman M. (2006). *Take a Nap! Change Your Life.* New York, NY: Workman Publishing Company, Inc.

Mesquita G, and Reimao R. (2010). Quality of sleep among university students: Effects of nighttime computer and television use. *Arquivos de Neuro-Psiquiatria* 68 (5): 720–725.

Milner CE, and Cote KA. (2009). Benefits of napping in healthy adults: Impact of nap length, time of day, age, and experience with napping. *Journal of Sleep Research* 18 (2) 272–281.

Morita E, Miyazaki S, and Okawa M. (2012). Pilot study on the effects of a 1-day sleep education program: Influence on sleep of stopping alcohol intake at bedtime. *Nagoya Journal of Medical Science* 74 (3–4): 359–365.

Myllymäki T, Kyröläinen H, Savolainen K, et al. (2011). Effects of vigorous late-night exercise on sleep quality and cardiac autonomic activity. *Journal of Sleep Research* 20 (1 Part 2): 146–153.

National Sleep Foundation. (2013). *Sleeping smart.* National Sleep Foundation. Retrieved on July 11, 2015 from www.sleepfoundation.org.

Prather AA, Janicki-Deverts D, Hall MH, et al. (2015). Behaviorally assessed sleep and susceptibility to the common cold. *SLEEP* 38 (9): 1353–1359.

Reid KJ, Baron KG, Lu B, et al. (2010). Aerobic exercise improves self-reported sleep and quality of life in older adults with insomnia. *Sleep Medicine* 11 (9): 934–940.

Sargent C, Lastella M, Halson SL, et al. (2014). The impact of training schedules on the sleep and fatigue of elite athletes. *Chronobiology International* 31 (10): 1160–1168.

Siengsukon CF, and Boyd LA. (2009). Does sleep promote motor learning? Implications for physical rehabilitation. *Physical Therapy* 89 (4): 370–383.

Stone KL, Ancoli-Israel S, Blackwell T, et al. (2008). Actigraphy-measured sleep characteristics and risk of falls in older women. *Archives of Internal Medicine* 168 (16): 1768–1775.

UCLA Conference. (2009). *Third Annual Advances in Sleep Medicine* (conference manual). Los Angeles, CA. February 21.

UCLA Conference. (2010). *Fourth Annual Sleep Medicine: A Practical Approach for Primary Care* (conference manual). Los Angeles, CA. September 25.

University of Michigan Health System (Dr. DA Williams and Dr. M Carey). (2003). Sleep Hygiene. Retrieved on July 11, 2015 from www.med.umich.edu/painresearch/patients/sleep.pdf.

Van Reen E, Tarokh L, Rupp TL, et al. (2011). Does timing of alcohol administration affect sleep? *Sleep* 34 (2): 195–205.

Walker MP. (2009). The role of sleep in cognition and emotion. *Annals of the New York Academy of Sciences* 1156: 168–197.

Wilk KE, and Joyner D. (2014). *The Use of Aquatics in Orthopedic and Sports Medicine Rehabilitation and Physical Conditioning.* Thorofare, NJ: SLACK.

Zee PC, and Goldstein CA. (2010). Treatment of shift work disorder and jet lag. *Current Treatment Options in Neurology* 12 (5): 396–411.

PART 3
Managing Your Stress

Some causes of stress include chronic overstimulation of the senses (excessive noise or overcrowding), lack of sleep, poor diet, overtraining with exercise, information overload (due to cellular phones and the Internet), constant barrage of conflict and bad news via various media outlets, financial concerns, relationship problems, or job issues.

Hans Selye, MD, PhD, an endocrinologist known for his research on the effects of stress on the human body, stated that "activity and rest must be judiciously balanced, and every person has his own characteristic requirements for rest and activity." Dr. Selye wrote three popular books (Selye 1974,1976,1976) on the subject.

Research says...

- A study by Widaman (2016) found that "Chronic stress was related to evening eating choices and overall empty calories in the diet of breakfast skippers."
- Stress and depression can promote obesity (Kiecolt-Glaser et al. 2015).
- Stress management for individuals with type 2 diabetes mellitus has a beneficial role for stress levels and glycemic control (Koloverou et al. 2014).
- Stress can accelerate cellular aging (Epel 2008).
- Stress can have harmful effects on the heart (Dimsdale 2008).
- Stress from hostile or abrasive relationships can affect physiological functioning and health dynamics such as wound healing (Kiecolt-Glaser et al. 2005).
- Stress can slow wound healing (Kiecolt-Glaser et al. 1995).

Use the following strategies to reduce your stress levels:

- Smile a lot! Smiling stretches the facial muscles and improves your mood (Abel 2002; Hess et al. 2001). Smile, and others will smile with you (Niedenthal 2007).
- Exercise. Go for a walk, hike, or bike ride.
- Take a yoga class (Kiecolt-Glaser et al. 2010).
- Try tai chi or qigong.
- Relax in a hammock under a shady tree.
- Engage in music, art, and hobbies.
- Play with your pets.
- Yawn while stretching your face and body as a wake-up cue or relaxation technique throughout the day. Some clinicians believe yawning might increase arousal (Gupta et al. 2013), while others feel it can reduce anger, anxiety, and stress.
- Try acupuncture.
- Get a massage or use self-massage to relax upper- and lower-body muscles.
- Close your eyes lightly for a 10-second mini-break after close-up work on a computer.
- Create a daily "to do" list each morning so you don't have to stress over having to remember simple things you need to take care of throughout your day.
- Use a reading stand while sitting in a chair or on a bed to relieve neck strain and shoulder tension.
- Try aromatherapy. The smells of lavender, rose, vanilla, and lemongrass can put you in a relaxed mood (Murad 2010).
- Try the Emotional Freedom Technique (EFT) (Church et al. 2012).
- Try attending a Japanese Tea Ceremony. An article by Keenan (1996) indicates that "Serious practitioners of tea develop a mind set and body control that enables them to transform tension-producing details of everyday life into moments of beauty, meaningfulness and tranquility." A study by Shiah et al. (2013) indicates that "Tea treated with good intentions improved mood more than ordinary tea derived from the same source."
- Reduce work (or school) stress by glancing away frequently from close visual tasks and training yourself to "look easy" to reduce physiological stress. To "look easy" simply means to keep your facial muscles, jaw, and mind relaxed enough to accomplish and concentrate on the task with ease and purpose (Birnbaum 1985).

- Go outside for a walk to get fresh air and natural light, and to look off into the distance. For example, look at the clouds, distant trees, or out over the ocean or lake without squinting. Gazing into the distance tends to relax while prolonged close-up work can lead to stress (Birnbaum 1984,1985).
- Keep forehead muscles relaxed. While on the phone or computer, periodically touch your forehead muscles to feel if they are activated. If eyebrows are raised or forehead crinkled, practice relaxing your facial muscles.
- Keep your jaw and mouth in a relaxed position. For a relaxed "neutral" jaw position, your mouth should be closed lightly with lips together and teeth not touching. Rest the upper part of the tip of your tongue against the hard palate just behind your upper central incisors. Breathe through your nose using diaphragmatic breathing (Hertling 2011; Rocabado et al. 1991).
- Relax in a reclining chair. This can relieve pressure on your low-back region. Or, relax in a rocking chair. A study shows that individuals with Alzheimer's disease who *actively* use a rocking chair for one to two hours per day show significant improvements in anxiety, depression, and balance, and also a reduction in pain medication usage (Pierce et al. 2009). Another study indicates that active rocking might be a good form of low-exertion exercise for frail, elderly individuals (Houston 1993).
- Limit unnecessary decision-making. An article by Vohs et al. (2008) indicates that "making choices led to reduced self-control (i.e., less physical stamina, reduced persistence in the face of failure, more procrastination, and less quality and quantity of arithmetic calculations)."
- Try providing a helping hand to those in need, but at some point consider distancing yourself from perpetually negative individuals.
- Stop relationships which are not going anywhere and bringing you down.
- Finally, think positive. Your body believes what your brain tells it.

References

Abel MH. (2002). *An Empirical Reflection on the Smile (Mellen Studies in Psychology* (Volume 4). Lewiston, NY: Edwin Mellen Press.

Birnbaum MH. (1984). Nearpoint visual stress: A physiological model. *Journal of the American Optometric Association* 55 (11): 825–835.

Birnbaum MH. (1985). Nearpoint visual stress: Clinical implications. *Journal of the American Optometric Association* 56 (6): 480–490.

Block SH, and Block CB. (2014). *Mind-Body Workbook for Anxiety: Effective Tools for Overcoming Panic, Fear, and Worry.* Oakland, CA: New Harbinger Publications, Inc.

Church D, Yount G, and Brooks AJ. (2012). The effect of emotional freedom techniques on stress biochemistry: A randomized controlled trial. *Journal of Nervous and Mental Disease* 200 (10): 891–896.

Dimsdale JE. (2008). Psychological stress and cardiovascular disease. *Journal of the American College of Cardiology* 51 (13): 1237–1246.

Epel ES. (2009). Psychological and metabolic stress: A recipe for accelerated cellular aging? *Hormones* 8 (1): 7–22.

Gupta S, and Mittal S. (2013). Yawning and its physiological significance. *International Journal of Applied & Basic Medical Research* 3 (1): 11–15.

Hertling D. (2011). The temporomandibular joint. In: Brody LT, and Hall CM. *Therapeutic Exercise: Moving Toward Function,* 3rd ed. Baltimore, MD: Lippincott Williams & Wilkins.

Hess U, and Blairy S. (2001). Facial mimicry and emotional contagion to dynamic emotional facial expressions and their influence on decoding accuracy. *International Journal of Psychophysiology* 40 (2): 129–141.

Houston KA. (1993). An investigation of rocking as relaxation for the elderly. Does rocking elicit in the elderly the physiologic changes of the relaxation response? *Geriatric Nursing* 14 (4): 186–189.

Keenan J. (1996). The Japanese Tea Ceremony and stress management. *Holistic Nursing Practice* 10 (2): 30–37.

Kiecolt-Glaser JK, Christian L, Preston H, et al. (2010). Stress, inflammation, and yoga practice. *Psychosomatic Medicine* 72 (2): 113–121.

Kiecolt-Glaser JK, Habash DL, Fagundes CP, et al. (2015). Daily stressors, past depression, and metabolic responses to high-fat meals: A novel path to obesity. *Biological Psychiatry* 77 (7): 653–660.

Kiecolt-Glaser JK, Loving TJ, Stowell JR, et al. (2005). Hostile marital interactions, proinflammatory cytokine production, and wound healing. *Archives General Psychiatry* 62 (12): 1377–1384.

Kiecolt-Glaser K, Marucha PT, Malarkey WB, et al. (1995). Slowing of wound healing by psychological stress. *Lancet* 346 (8984): 1194–1196.

Koloverou E, Tentolouris N, Bakoula C, et al. (2014). Implementation of a stress management program in outpatients with type 2 diabetes mellitus: A randomized controlled trial. *Hormones (Athens, Greece)* 13 (4): 509–518.

Murad H. (2010). *The Water Secret: The Cellular Breakthrough to Look and Feel 10 Years Younger*. Hoboken, NJ: John Wiley & Sons, Inc.

Niedenthal, PM. (2007). Embodying emotion. *Science* 316 (5827): 1002–1005.

Pierce C, Pecen J, and McLeod KJ. (2009). Influence of seated rocking on blood pressure in the elderly: A pilot clinical study. *Biological Research for Nursing* 11 (2): 144–151.

Rocabado M, and Iglarsh ZA. (1991). *Musculoskeletal Approach to Maxillofacial Pain*. Philadelphia, PA: JB Lippincott.

Sapolsky RM. (2004). *Why Zebras Don't Get Ulcers: The Acclaimed Guide to Stress, Stress-Related Diseases, and Coping*, 3rd ed. New York, NY: St Martin's Griffin.

Selye H. (1974). *Stress without Distress*. Philadelphia, PA: Lippincott.

Selye H. (1976). *Stress in Health and Disease*. Boston, MA: Butterworths.

Selye H. (1976). *The Stress of Life*, revised edition. New York, NY: McGraw-Hill.

Shiah YJ, and Radin D. (2013). Metaphysics of the tea ceremony: A randomized trial investigating the roles of intention and belief on mood while drinking tea. *Explore (NY)* 9 (6): 355–360.

Vohs KD, Baumeister RF, Schmeichel BJ, et al. (2008). Making choices impairs subsequent self-control: a limited-resource account of decision making, self-regulation, and active initiative. *Journal of Personality and Social Psychology* 94 (5): 883–898.

Widaman AM, Witbracht MG, Forester SM, et al. (2016). Chronic stress is associated with indicators of diet quality in habitual breakfast skippers. *Journal of the Academy of Nutrition and Dietetics* 116 (11): 1776-1784.

PART 4
Nutrition for Life

Note: please speak with a registered dietitian to obtain specific nutritional guidelines for your needs. The following is not intended to be a complete coverage of nutrition information. Instead the focus is on some of the health benefits of fruits and vegetables to inspire individuals to include more of these in their diets.

Mindful Eating

A study by Miller et al. (2014) states that "mindful eating may be an effective intervention for increasing awareness of hunger and satiety cues, improving eating regulation and dietary patterns, reducing symptoms of depression and anxiety, and promoting weight loss." Consider the following cues to include mindful eating as a part of your meals:

- Avoid emotional eating.
- Sit in a firm and supportive chair.
- Turn off all electronic devices.
- Avoid talking while chewing your food to not only enjoy the satisfying tastes, but also to prevent choking.
- Chew your food slowly.
- Sit in a location that allows you to look at nature or pleasant scenery.
- Avoid discussing business or personal problems while eating to allow for digestion.

Engage your five senses:

- **Observe** the colors in your food (such as the red, orange, green, and yellow colors).

- **Feel** your food's textures (the shape of a berry or carrot).
- **Listen** to sounds your foods make (the crunching of celery or an apple).
- **Smell** your food's delicious aromas (the scent of mint or cinnamon).
- **Taste** the sweet, salty, bitter, sour, or spice in your foods (such as the tartness of a lemon)

You Cannot Outrun A Bad Diet

An editorial article by Malhotra et al. (2015) states that "It is time to wind back the harms caused by the junk food industry's Public Relations machinery. Let us bust the myth of physical inactivity and obesity. You cannot outrun a bad diet."

What Foods Should I Choose?

Good nutrition is a balance of healthful proteins (such as fish, grass-fed beef or lamb, chicken, yogurt, cheese, nuts, seeds, or legumes), healthful fats (such as nuts, seeds, olive oil, or avocados), healthful carbohydrates (such as vegetables, fruits, or whole grains), and healthful beverages (such as water or tea). The following sections also focus on guidelines to help you fine-tune choices during grocery trips.

Practical Nutrition

Consider looking at nutrition this way: Could you pick or catch the foods you are currently eating? In other words, could you have picked that box of cookies from a tree or caught those doughnuts fishing in a lake or ocean? The best wholesome foods for your body will typically be those that give you enough calories, allow your body to heal and maintain itself, and do not cause stomach irritation, nausea, cramping, bloating, or allergies. The more you speak with people around you, it becomes apparent that almost any food can cause an adverse reaction in someone. Therefore, the right food choices for each individual are critical for optimal health.

Individual dietary choices are influenced by habits, culture, nutritional knowledge, price, availability, taste, and convenience. A study by Imamura et al. (2015) systematically assessed different dietary patterns across 187 nations in 1990 and 2010 and the authors conclude that "Increases in unhealthy patterns are outpacing increases in healthy patterns in most world regions." Our multicultural and global society needs to find ways to reduce the financial barriers to healthful eating, which in turn can reduce illness and disease (Rao et al. 2013). Also, food is not only important for human health, but health of the planet since agriculture impacts environmental sustainability (Tilman et al. 2014).

Also, a person can eat in a healthful manner whether he or she is a vegetarian or a nonvegetarian. Healthfully eating can come in a variety of packages. The key to good nutrition is not only choosing foods that agree with your body, but selecting foods that are processed as little as possible and closest to the way nature intends for us to eat.

Choosing Wisely

Every purchase we make or don't make influences the marketplace. If a significant percentage of the population chose healthful foods and snacks, then the fast-food, soft drink, and junk food industries would eventually either have to change their approach or become obsolete. After all, "we are what we eat." Ideally, consider choosing quality foods which adhere to the following fresh farm-to-table approach:

- Produced as eco-friendly and with recyclable materials
- Produced in a sustainable manner
- Product claims are 100% truthful
- Product is truly all-natural
- Free of genetically modified organisms (GMO-free)
- Antibiotic-free
- Pesticide-, additive- and chemical-free
- Free of artificial colors, flavors, sweeteners, or preservatives
- Free of artificial growth hormones
- Locally grown
- Organic
- Animals are cage-free (chicken and eggs)
- Animals are free-range and grass-fed
- Fish are wild caught

For additional good health, try the following:

- Shop at farmer's markets
- Eat a variety of colors and seasonal fruits and vegetables
- Eat in moderate amounts
- Eat slow

We all know good nutrition is not about "cookies and cakes and pies, oh my!" A calorie is not just a calorie. Your source of food has a tremendous impact on your health. Calories from doughnuts do not carry the same life-sustaining nutrients as berries or green leafy vegetables. The calories might be the same, but nutritional content and the life-giving effect is not.

Proper nutrition should be an accessible concept available to all groups of people. Everyone can eat healthfully without spending tons of money on supplements and specialized foods. Supplements typically come in handy when there is a deficiency or some specific need, such as low levels of calcium or vitamin D. Nourish yourself with food first, and then supplement only if necessary.

Research says…

- The Mediterranean diet "decreases inflammation and improves endothelial function" (Schwingshackl et al. 2014).
- A traditional Mediterranean diet "could modify markers of heart failure toward a more protective mode" (Fito et al. 2014).
- "A Paleolithic diet improved glycemic control and several cardiovascular risk factors compared to a diabetes diet in patients with type 2 diabetes" (Jonsson et al. 2013).
- "A low-fat plant-based diet in a corporate setting improved body weight, plasma lipids, and, in individuals with diabetes, glycemic control" (Mishra et al. 2013).
- A study called the Dietary Approaches to Stop Hypertension (DASH) indicates that individuals with hypertension can lower their blood pressure through lifestyle and behavioral changes consisting of weight loss, sodium reduction, increased physical activity, and limited alcohol consumption (Appel et al. 2003).

Food Allergies and Sensitivities
Specialized diets might also come into play for individuals with certain medical conditions (such as diabetes or hypertension), celiac disease (gluten allergy), food allergies (such as to eggs, fish, shellfish, soy, peanuts, tree nuts, or milk), or food intolerances (such as lactose or fructose) and sensitivities (such as to additives, preservatives, corn, or yeast).

Finding Your Ideal Diet
There are *hundreds* of good, informative nutrition books in the marketplace. What disappoints many individuals is that not all concepts and strategies work for everyone.

The same holds true for exercise concepts and training methods. This is why so many diet and exercise programs fail. Explore many different strategies until you find a healthy one that works for you.

Rather than drawing swords, focus on self-discovery for improving health. For different perspectives, look through a variety of nutrition books and discuss them with your healthcare provider and dietitian. Find the approach that fits your needs.

Phytonutrients and Your Health

Eating 400 grams to 600 grams (which is equivalent to approximately three to four medium-sized apples) a day of fruits and vegetables is associated with reduced incidence of various forms of cancer, heart disease, and many chronic diseases (Heber et al. 2006; Pennington et al. 2010). This is consistent with the recommendation of the World Health Organization that increasing individual fruit and vegetable consumption to approximately 600 grams per day could reduce ischemic stroke worldwide (Lock et al. 2005).

In the book *What Color Is Your Diet?*, David Heber, MD, PhD, and Susan Bowerman, MS, RD, state that "foods can be classified according to color—red, red/purple, orange, orange/yellow, green, yellow/green, and white/green—based on the specific chemicals that absorb light in the visible spectrum and thus create the different colors. These chemicals are called 'phytonutrients' or 'phytochemicals,' and each of these colored compounds works in different ways to protect your genes and your DNA." The authors further state that "there are 150,000 edible plant species on earth, and we have just listed about 60 or so varieties in our Color Code. While this is a big improvement over the few servings per day the average American eats, there is still a long way to go to get to the over 800 varieties eaten by hunter-gatherers."

The Rainbow Nutrition Guide (see Table 1) outlines one way to organize your eating plan so you include more healthful fruits and vegetables into your diet. Why eat all this variety? Look at it like this: You are simply stacking the odds in your favor for maintaining good health. However, keep in mind what health author and registered dietitian Tracy Olgeaty Gensler MS, RD (Altug and Gensler 2006), states that "While it's tempting to champion the well-researched fruits or vegetables over the others, every single fruit and vegetable offers you some health benefit."

Table 1. Rainbow Nutrition Guide

Groups	Compounds	Some Research Areas	Food Sources
Green Group	sulforaphane, isothiocyanate, indole	Sulforaphane inhibits breast cancer stem cells (Li et al. 2010) Broccoli may reduce risk of prostate cancer (Traka et al. 2008)	• bok choy, broccoli, Brussels sprouts, cabbage, Chinese cabbage, kale, watercress
Yellow/Green Group	lutein, zeaxanthin	Lutein and zeaxanthin have a potential role in the prevention and treatment of certain eye diseases, such as age-related macular degeneration, cataract, and retinitis pigmentosa (Ma et al. 2010)	• avocado, collard greens, green beans, green peas, green and yellow peppers, mustard greens, romaine lettuce, spinach, turnip greens, yellow corn, zucchini • honeydew melon, kiwifruit
White/Green Group	allyl sulfide (allicin), flavonoid (quercetin and kaempferol	Has antibacterial, antiviral, and antitumor effects (Heber 2001; Venes 2013) Lowers blood cholesterol levels (Venes 2013) Garlic-derived compounds are effective to inhibit a variety of human cancers, such as prostate, breast, colon, skin, lung, and bladder cancers (Wang et al. 2010)	• asparagus, celery, chives, endive, garlic, leek, mushroom, onion, shallot • pear
Orange/Yellow Group	beta-cryptoxanthin	Helps fight heart disease Fruits high in antioxidant nutrients appear to be associated with reduced risk of incident squamous intraepithelial lesions of the cervix (Siegel et al. 2010)	• guava, kumquat, nectarine, orange, papaya, peach, pineapple, star fruit, tangelo, tangerine
Orange Group	alpha- and beta-carotene	A diet rich in beta-carotene and lutein/zeaxanthin may play a role in renal cell carcinoma prevention (Hu et al. 2009) Beta-carotene and lycopene were associated with a lower prevalence of metabolic syndrome (Sluijs et al. 2009)	• acorn squash, butternut squash, carrot, orange pepper, pumpkin, sweet potato, winter squash, yellow squash • apricot, cantaloupe, mango, persimmon
Red Group	lycopene	Can protect the cells in the body from oxidative damage Lycopene inhibits in vitro cell growth and induces apoptosis (programmed cell death) in breast and prostate cancer cells (Gullett et al. 2010)	• pink grapefruit, pink grapefruit juice, tomato (cooked and raw), tomato juice, tomato paste, tomato sauce, tomato soup, watermelon
Red/Purple Group	anthocyanin	May have a beneficial effect on heart disease by inhibiting blood clot formation and are anti-inflammatory (Heber 2001) May help with age-related declines in mental function Pomegranate may retard prostate cancer progression and inhibit growth of breast cancer cells (Gullett et al. 2010)	• cooked beets, purple cabbage • blackberry, blueberry, cherry, cranberry, cranberry juice, cranberry sauce, fig, grape juice, pear, plum, pomegranate, prune, purple passion fruit, raspberry, red apple, red grapes, strawberry

Adapted from Heber D, and Bowerman S. (2001). *What Color is Your Diet?* New York: Harper Collins/Regan; Altug and Gensler 2006; Heber et al. 2006; Steinmetz et al. 1991, 1991, 1996.

Reasoning for Seasoning

A variety of spices have been shown to help inflammatory diseases such as cancer, atherosclerosis, myocardial infarction, diabetes, allergy, asthma, arthritis, Crohn's disease, multiple sclerosis, Alzheimer's disease, osteoporosis, psoriasis, septic shock, and AIDS (Aggarwal et al. 2004, 2008).

An article by Gupta et al. (2010) states that "the human body consists of about 13 trillion cells, almost all of which are turned over within 100 days, indicating that 70,000 cells undergo apoptosis (programmed cell death) every minute. Thus, apoptosis/cell death is a normal physiological process." They further state "It is now believed that 90 percent to 95 percent of all cancers are attributed to lifestyle, with the remaining 5 percent to 10 percent attributed to faulty genes."

The medical profession is now turning its focus to the use of plant-derived dietary agents called nutraceuticals. We know that pharmaceuticals pertain to drugs or the pharmacy. The authors of this article explain that "A nutraceutical (a term formed by combining the words 'nutrition' and 'pharmaceutical') is simply any substance considered to be a food or part of a food that provides medical and health benefits."

Another article discusses nutraceuticals such as curcumin, carotenoids, acetyl-L-carnitine, coenzyme Q_{10}, vitamin D, and polyphenols, all natural substances that might help reduce the expression of disease-promoting genes (Virmani et al. 2013). Perhaps very soon, all major supermarkets will display the healing and prevention properties, based on research, of every single fruit and vegetable in the store.

The Foods and Spices Guide (see Table 2) helps you understand the benefits of various compounds. Always consult with your physician or healthcare provider before using spices, herbs, or supplements for medical purposes. If you take medications, there could be adverse reactions (Stargrove et al. 2008).

Additional Resources

- American Botanical Council, www.abc.herbalgram.org
- Herb Research Foundation, www.herbs.org
- HerbMed, www.herbmed.org

Table 2. Foods and Spices Guide		
Food Source	**Active Compound**	**Some Areas of Benefit**
Aloe	Emodin	Antioxidant, anti-inflammatory, antifungal, immunoprotective (El-Shemy et al. 2010)
Basil and rosemary	Ursolic acid	Chemopreventive activity (Aggarwal et al. 2004)
Black pepper	Piper nigrum	Anti-inflammatory, antioxidant, and anticancer activities (Liu et al. 2010)
Cloves	Eugenol	Antioxidant and anti-inflammatory activities (Aggarwal et al. 2004)
Fennel, anise, coriander	Anethol	Antioxidant and anti-inflammatory activities (Aggarwal et al. 2004)
Garlic	Diallyl sulfide, ajoene, S-ally cysteine, allicin	Chemopreventive and anti-inflammatory activities (Aggarwal et al. 2004; Mehta et al. 2010)
Ginger	Gingerol	Chemopreventive potential, treatment of nausea with motion or chemotherapy, anti-inflammatory (Aggarwal et al. 2004; Mehta et al. 2010)
Gingko biloba	Ginkgolides	Chemoprevention, antioxidant, anti-inflammatory activities (Mehta et al. 2010; Ye et al. 2007)
Ginseng	Ginsenoside	Antiviral against influenza A virus (Lee et al. 2014)
Green tea	Catechins	Chemopreventive potential (Gullett et al. 2010)
Honey-bee propolis	Caffeic acid	Anti-inflammatory and antimicrobial effects (Khayyal et al.1993; Sherlock et al. 2010)
Oleander	Oleanderin	Chemopreventive potential (Afaq et al. 2004)
Parsley	Apigenin	Antioxidant capacity (Henning et al. 2011; Meeran et al. 2008)
Red chili pepper	Capsaicin	Chemopreventive potential (Aggarwal et al. 2004)
Soybean	Genistein	Antioxidant (Gullett et al. 2010)
Sumac (spice)	Rhus coriaria	Hypoglycemic and antioxidant activity (Candan et al. 2004; Giancarlo et al. 2006)
Turmeric	Curcumin	Chemopreventive, anti-inflammatory, lowers blood cholesterol, improves arthritis associated symptoms (Aggarwal et al. 2004; Gullett et al. 2010; Panahi et al. 2014)

References

Afaq F, Saleem M, Aziz MH, et al. (2004). Inhibition of 12-O-tetradecanoylphorbol-13-acetate-induced tumor promotion markers in CD-1 mouse skin by oleandrin. *Toxicology and Applied Pharmacology* 195 (3): 361–369.

Aggarwal BB, Kunnumakkara AB, Harikumar KB, et al. (2008). Potential of spice-derived phytochemicals for cancer prevention. *Planta Medica* 74 (13): 1560–1569.

Aggarwal BB, and Shishodia S. (2004). Suppression of nuclear factor-kappa B activation pathway by spice-derived phytochemicals: Reasoning for seasoning. *Annals of the New York Academy of Sciences* 1030: 434–441.

Altug Z, and Gensler TO. (2006). *The Anti-Aging Fitness Prescription: A Day-by-Day Nutrition and Workout Plan to Age-Proof Your Body and Mind.* New York, NY: Healthy Living Books.

Appel LJ, Champagne CM, Harsha DW, et al. (2003). Effects of comprehensive lifestyle modification on blood pressure control: Main results of the premier clinical trial. *JAMA* 289 (16): 2083–2093.

Candan F, and Sokmen A. (2004). Effects of Rhus coriaria L (Anacardiaceae) on lipid peroxidation and free radical scavenging activity. *Phytotherapy Research* 18 (1): 84–86.

Clark N. (2014). *Nancy Clark's Sports Nutrition Guidebook*, 5th ed. Champaign IL: Human Kinetics.

Cordain L. (2010). The Paleo Diet, revised edition. Hoboken, NJ: John Wiley & Sons, Inc.

Cullum-Dugan D, and Pawlak R. (2015). Position of the academy of nutrition and dietetics: Vegetarian diets. *Journal of the Academy of Nutrition and Dietetics* 115 (5): 801–810. www.andjrnl.org/article/S2212-2672%2815%2900261-0/pdf.

Duyff RL. (2012). The American Dietetic Association's Complete Food & Nutrition Guide, 4th ed. New York, NY: Houghton Mifflin Harcourt Publishing Company.

El-Shemy HA, Aboul-Soud MA, Nassr-Allah AA, et al. (2010). Antitumor properties and modulation of antioxidant enzymes' activity by aloe vera leaf active principles isolated via supercritical carbon dioxide extraction. *Current Medicinal Chemistry* 17 (2): 129–138.

Fito M, Estruch R, Salas-Salvado J, et al. (2014). Effect of the Mediterranean diet on heart failure biomarkers: A randomized sample from the PREDIMED trial. *European Journal of Heart Failure* 16 (5): 543–550.

Fuhrman J. (2011). Eat to Live: The Amazing Nutrient Rich Program for Fast and Sustained Weight Loss. New York, NY: Little, Brown and Company.

Giancarlo S, Rosa LM, Nadjafi F, et al. (2006). Hypoglycaemic activity of two spices extracts: Rhus coriaria L. and Bunium persicum Boiss. *Natural Product Research* 20 (9): 882–886.

Gullett NP, Amin ARMR, Bayraktar S, et al. (2010). Cancer prevention with natural compounds. *Seminars in Oncology* 37 (3): 258–281.

Gupta SC, Kim JH, Prasad S, et al. (2010). Regulation of survival, proliferation, invasion, angiogenesis, and metastasis of tumor cells through modulation of inflammatory pathways by nutraceuticals. *Cancer and Metastasis Reviews* 29 (3): 405–434.

Heber D, Blackburn GL, Go VLW, et al. (Eds.). (2006). *Nutritional Oncology*, 2nd ed. Boston, MA: Academic Press.

Heber D, and Bowerman S. (2001). *What Color is Your Diet?* New York, NY: HarperCollins.

Henning SM, Zhang Y, Seeram NP, et al. (2011). Antioxidant capacity and phyto-chemical content of herbs and spices in dry, fresh and blended herb paste form. *International Journal of Food Sciences and Nutrition* 62 (3): 219–225.

Hu J, La Vecchia C, Negri E, et al. (2009). Dietary vitamin C, E, and carotenoid intake and risk of renal cell carcinoma. *Cancer Causes & Control* 20 (8): 1451–1458.

Imamura F, Micha R, Khatibzadeh S, et al. (2015). Dietary quality among men and women in 187 countries in 1990 and 2010: A systematic assessment. *Lancet. Global Health* 3 (3): e132–142.

James JM, Burks W, and Eigenmann P. (2012). *Food Allergy*. St. Louis, MO: Elsevier Saunders.

Jonsson T, Granfeldt Y, Ahren B, et al. (2009). Beneficial effects of a Paleolithic diet on cardiovascular risk factors in type 2 diabetes: A randomized cross-over pilot study. *Cardiovascular Diabetology* 8: 35.

Kohn JB. (2014). Is there a diet for histamine intolerance? *Journal of the Academy of Nutrition and Dietetics* 114 (11): 1860.

Khayyal MT, el-Ghazaly MA, and el-Khatib AS. (1993). Mechanisms involved in the anti-inflammatory effect of propolis extract. *Drugs under Experimental and Clinical Research* 19 (5): 197–203.

Lee JS, Hwang HS, Ko EJ, et al. (2014). Immunomodulatory activity of red ginseng against influenza A virus infection. *Nutrients* 6 (2): 517–529.

Li Y, Zhang T, Korkaya H, et al. (2010). Sulforaphane, a dietary component of broccoli/broccoli sprouts, inhibits breast cancer stem cells. *Clinical Cancer Research* 16 (9): 2580–2590.

Liu Y, Yadev VR, Aggarwal BB, et al. (2010). Inhibitory effects of black pepper (Piper nigrum) extracts and compounds on human tumor cell proliferation, cyclooxygenase enzymes, lipid peroxidation and nuclear transcription factor-kappa-B. *Natural Product Communications* 5 (8): 1253–1257.

Lock K, Pomerleau J, Causer L, et al. (2005). The global burden of disease attributable to low consumption of fruit and vegetables: Implications for the global strategy on diet. *Bulletin of the World Health Organization* 83: 100–108.

Ma L, and Lin XM. (2010). Effects of lutein and zeaxanthin on aspects of eye health. *Journal of the Science of Food and Agriculture* 90 (1): 2–12.

Mahan LK, Escott-Stump S, and Raymond JL. (2012). *Krause's Food and the Nutrition Care Process*, 13th ed. St. Louis, MO: Elsevier Sanders.

Meeran SM, and Katiyar SK. (2008). Cell cycle control as a basis for cancer chemoprevention through dietary agents. *Frontiers in Bioscience* 13: 2191–2202.

Mehta RG, Murillo G, Naithani R, et al. (2010). Cancer chemoprevention by natural products: How far have we come? *Pharmaceutical Research* 27 (6): 950–961.

Mishra S, Xu J, Agarwal U, et al. (2013). A multicenter randomized controlled trial of a plant-based nutrition program to reduce body weight and cardiovascular risk in the corporate setting: The GEICO study. *European Journal of Clinical Nutrition* 67 (7): 718–724.

Panahi Y, Rahimnia AR, Sharafi M, et al. (2014). Curcuminoid treatment for knee osteoarthritis: A randomized double-blind placebo-controlled trial. *Phytotherapy Research* 28 (11): 1625–1631.

Pennington JAT, and Spungen J. (2010). *Bowes & Church's Food Values of Portions Commonly Used*, 19th ed. Baltimore, MD: Lippincott Williams & Wilkins.

Pollan M. (2008). *In Defense of Food: An Eater's Manifesto.* New, NY: Penguin Press.

Rao M, Afshin A, Singh G, et al. (2013). Do healthier foods and diet patterns cost more than less healthy options? A systematic review and meta-analysis. *BMJ Open* 3 (12): e004277.

Schwingshackl L, and Hoffmann G. (2014). Mediterranean dietary pattern, inflammation and endothelial function: A systematic review and meta-analysis of intervention trials. *Nutrition, Metabolism & Cardiovascular Diseases* 24 (9): 929–939.

Shanahan C, and Shanahan L. (2009). *Deep Nutrition: Why Your Genes Need Traditional Food.* Lawai, HI: Big Box Books.

Sherlock O, Dolan A, Athman R, et al. (2010). Comparison of the antimicrobial activity of Ulmo honey from Chile and Manuka honey against methicillin-resistant Staphylococcus aureus, Escherichia coli and Pseudomonas aeruginosa. *BMC Complementary and Alternative Medicine* 10: 47.

Siegel EM, Salemi JL, Villa LL, et al. (2010). Dietary consumption of antioxidant nutrients and risk of incident cervical intraepithelial neoplasia. *Gynecologic Oncology* 118 (3): 289–294.

Sluijs I, Beulens JW, Grobbee DE, et al. (2009). Dietary carotenoid intake is associated with lower prevalence of metabolic syndrome in middle-aged and elderly men. *Journal of Nutrition* 139 (5): 987–992.

Stargrove M, Treasure J, and McKee D. (2008). *Herb, Nutrient, and Drug Interactions: Clinical Implications and Therapeutic Strategies.* St. Louis, MO: Mosby Elsevier.

Steinmetz KA, and Potter JD. (1991). Vegetables, fruit, and cancer. I. Epidemiology. *Cancer Causes & Control* 2 (5): 325–357.

Steinmetz KA, and Potter JD. (1991). Vegetables, fruit, and cancer. II. Mechanisms. *Cancer Causes & Control* 2 (6): 427–442.

Steinmetz KA, and Potter JD. (1996). Vegetables, fruit, and cancer prevention: A review. *Journal of the American Dietetic Association* 96 (10): 1027–1039.

Tilman D, and Clark M. (2014). Global diets link environmental sustainability and human health. *Nature* 515: 518–522.

Traka M, Gasper AV, Melchini A, et al. (2008). Broccoli consumption interacts with GSTM1 to perturb oncogenic signaling pathways in the prostate. *PloS One* 3 (7): e2568.

Venes D. (Ed.) (2013). *Taber's Cyclopedic Medical Dictionary*, 22nd ed. Philadelphia, PA: FA Davis.

Villacorta M. (2013). *Peruvian Power Foods*. Deerfield, FL: Health Communications, Inc.

Virmani A, Pinto L, Binienda Z, et al. (2013). Food, nutrigenomics, and neurodegeneration-neuroprotection by what you eat! *Molecular Neurobiology* 48 (2): 353–362.

Wang YB, Qin J, Zheng XY, et al. (2010). Diallyl trisulfide induces Bcl-2 and caspase-3-dependent apoptosis via downregulation of Akt phosphorylation in human T24 bladder cancer cells. *Phytomedicine* 17 (5): 363–368.

Ye B, Aponte M, Dai Y, et al. (2007). Ginkgo biloba and ovarian cancer prevention: Epidemiological and biological evidence. *Cancer Letters* 251 (1): 43–52.

PART 5
Sustainable Exercise

Benefits of Exercise

Evidence-based exercise can be used therapeutically to improve activities of daily living, quality of life, and conditions such as osteoporosis, osteoarthritis, diabetes, hypertension, scoliosis, low back pain, and obesity. The following are some of the benefits of exercise:

- Increases endurance (stamina) and strength
- Reduces stress, anxiety, and depression
- Decreases blood pressure
- Lowers low-density lipoprotein (LDL) cholesterol (read: bad cholesterol)
- Raises high-density lipoprotein (HDL) cholesterol (read: good cholesterol)
- Improves sleep
- Improves control of blood sugar levels
- Improves flexibility, balance, coordination, agility, and reaction time
- Improves mood, self-confidence, cognitive processing speed, and attention span
- Improves posture and daily function (such as the ability to get out of a chair with ease)
- Improves pelvic floor strengthening before and after pregnancy
- Improvement in musculoskeletal issues (for example, less knee or shoulder pain)
- Improvement after orthopedic surgery, such as after total knee or hip replacement surgery, rotator cuff surgery, or back and neck surgery

- Improvement and control of medical conditions, such as asthma, diabetes, facial palsy, stroke, or peripheral neuropathy
- Alleviates back pain, especially when associated with decreased body weight
- Slows age-related decline in bone mineral density and improves bone density
- Slows age-related decline in muscle mass and strength, as well as improves muscle mass and strength
- Less risk of falling
- Less body fat and excess weight

Lifestyle and Functional Exercise

Lifestyle exercise is the performance of daily routine activities such as chores, errands, work, or hobbies. Functional exercise includes activities like rolling side to side in bed, moving from sitting in a chair to standing, squatting to lift a package, or carrying groceries. Here are some suggestions for increasing lifestyle and functional exercise:

- Park your car in the spot farthest from the store each time you shop.
- Take the stairs at work instead of the elevator.
- Walk to and from work if you live close enough.
- If you can, ride your bicycle to work or part of the way.
- While you watch your favorite television show, walk in place instead of sitting on the couch.
- Work in your garden.
- Vacuum the house.
- Rake leaves.
- Sweep the floor.
- Wash and vacuum your car.
- Walk up and down all the aisles in the grocery store before you shop.
- Walk while meeting with a work colleague.
- Walk around the mall from one end to the other before or after shopping.
- Walk to pick up lunch at work instead of ordering delivery.
- Take breaks at work and walk around the office from one end to the other.
- Walk once around the block before entering your house or apartment building.
- Take your dog for a walk, or take a walk with another best friend.

Exercise Guidelines

Please be aware that this section outlines some of my humble (and perhaps biased) opinions for training. When beginning a fitness routine, most people ask the following questions:

- "How many days a week should I train?"
- "How much weight should I use?"
- "How many sets or reps should I perform?"
- "How much rest should I take between sets and workouts?"

The answer to all of the above questions is this: It depends. There are no magic formulas—only guidelines. These statements refer to general fitness, but the same holds true for elite athletes in a variety of sports. Each person is unique and requires different movements at varied intervals. A football player does not train the same way a tennis player or swimmer trains. There are similar training strategies, but workouts are completely different to accommodate varied demands.

Training for fitness is different for each person and should be based on the following:

- What is the person's level of experience—beginner, intermediate, or advanced?
- How well does the person feel on training day?
- How much rest did the person get the previous night?
- How well-nourished and hydrated is the person on training day?
- Is the person mentally focused, or are there distractions?

There's also no rule that says every workout should be the same. Train with variety, and train to feel good—not to tear yourself down.

21 Body Rules for Exercising

This section outlines basic concepts to keep in mind when performing exercises. I take no credit for coming up with the body "rules" since top clinicians, trainers, and coaches have been using these principles for many years.

Many of these rules might not apply to elite athletes, who take risks and push the limits of their bodies for purposes of competition. If your primary goal is improving or maintaining good health or you are not an elite athlete, don't think about training like one. Instead focus on good health and keeping your body fit and mobile.

Activity is for everyone, from young to old. A study by Pahor et al. (2014) indicates that "a structured, moderate-intensity physical activity program compared with a health education program reduced major mobility disability over 2.6 years among older adults at risk for disability. These findings suggest mobility benefit from such a program in vulnerable older adults." The physical activity in this study included walking, and also strength, flexibility, and balance training.

I suggest you keep the following body "rules" in mind as you exercise:

RULE 1: FIRST DO NO HARM

Hippocrates, an ancient Greek physician known as the "father of medicine" (Venes 2013), is reported to have said, "First do no harm." Exercise is meant to make you feel better and improve your body and mind. The purpose of exercise is not to create injury or pain. Therefore, train without pain.

RULE 2: LISTEN TO YOUR BODY

Take your time figuring out which movements are best for your body. For example, some people might not be able to squat deeply due to their hip joint structure and soft-tissue limitations. You might need a wide squat stance while your workout partner does better with a narrow stance. Learn the natural patterns of your body.

RULE 3: RESPECT PAIN AND ITS SYMPTOMS

Be mindful of your body's signals. If an exercise hurts, modify it to a pain-free motion or skip it. Take charge of your pain by knowing which movements create discomfort and modifying activities and motions as necessary. Also, avoid movements and exercises that cause burning, tingling, numbness, and shooting or radiating pain.

RULE 4: THINK AND MOVE

Think about the movements as you perform a skill or activity.

RULE 5: TRAIN YOUR BRAIN

Mentally practicing a task or skill without actually doing the movement or exercise might help your body perform better.

RULE 6: SLOW DOWN

Consider not training with weights or body weight exercises when you are in a rush to finish or are distracted with other personal matters. Injuries can happen when you are in a hurry or not focused.

RULE 7: UNDERSTAND RISK VERSUS REWARD

Minimize or avoid risky exercises. Once again, if you are an elite athlete, there are certain assumed risks with training and competition. If not, then why risk breaks, tears, and injury? Train for longevity and sustainability.

RULE 8: DON'T OVERTRAIN

Exercise just enough to get good results, but don't overtrain.

RULE 9: BE AWARE OF YOUR POSTURE

Train with good form and body awareness to build and maintain good posture.

RULE 10: FOCUS ON FORM

Train with good form, and think about your movement patterns so you imprint these into your brain.

RULE 11: BREATHE PROPERLY

Breathe freely, even when you are stiffening your core muscles during exercises such as push-ups and squats.

RULE 12: SPARE YOUR SPINE

Stiffen your core muscles only enough for the task at hand. Professor Stuart McGill, PhD, states that "It takes sufficient stability and no more" (McGill 2014). If you are lifting a pencil off the ground, you will stiffen your core some but not maximally. However, if you are bending to lift and carry two heavy suitcases, you will stiffen the core to a much higher degree. How hard? It depends. It takes practice to determine how much you can lift and carry in real life or during exercise. Professional weight lifters take many years to learn how to safely lift, pull, push, and carry heavy loads. Go slow, and learn the limitations of your body. Also, protect your spine during exercise by maintaining the normal spine curves.

RULE 13: RECOVER AND RECUPERATE

Rest and recover thoroughly after workouts. Stay clear of training approaches that constantly push you and tear you down without respecting pain, recovery, and meaningful progress. Listen to your body. Also, periodically take time off from training to allow your body to fully recuperate from repetitive movements. This includes getting enough sleep every night. Even a good thing like exercise can be done in excess, so breaks are needed. After an extended vacation of one to four weeks, consider backing off to body weight exercises (meaning no additional resistance) for your strength workouts and cut back to around half the intensity on your other training. This allows your mind and body to ease back into your daily schedule.

RULE 14: TRAIN WITH VARIETY
Vary workouts to prevent injury and mental burnout. Don't get focused on one type of training.

RULE 15: BE ADAPTABLE
No two days are the same in a person's life. Modify your exercise routine (and nutrition program) when you have illness, pain, injury, excess stress levels, restricted sleep, or surgery.

RULE 16: BE OPEN-MINDED
Sports medicine and sports performance research continues to evolve. Researchers and clinicians are constantly finding new ways to make exercise, fitness, and sports conditioning safer and more effective. Stay abreast of the latest information.

RULE 17: MONITOR YOUR TRAINING LOAD
Discuss with your fitness professional or healthcare provider ways you can monitor your exercise and training loads to prevent injury. For example, you might use methods such as heart rate, blood pressure, rating of perceived exertion (RPE), and also questionnaires, diaries, and journals (Halson 2014).

RULE 18: CONTROL YOUR MENTAL STRESS
Uncontrolled stress can sap your energy and delay healing.

RULE 19: NOURISH YOUR BODY
Provide your body with needed nutrients for repair and maintenance before, during, and after workouts.

RULE 20: INCLUDE SOME ROTATIONAL EXERCISES
Include some rotational movement into your workouts since sports (such as golf, tennis, and basketball) and daily activities (such as reaching overhead or bending to tie your shoe) involve rotation of various body regions. Try rotational activities such as yoga, tai chi, qigong, or other martial arts.

RULE 21: SIMPLIFY

Even some strength and conditioning professionals who work with elite athletes question the current trend of overtraining and high-risk exercises. But trends come and go, and this one is changing not only in the athletic population, but also in the general fitness population, with the focus now centering on the least amount of training for maximum results. If five exercises give you the same results as 10, which program would you choose? Choosing the five-exercise program is a no-brainer. It's all about precision training versus a shotgun approach.

Did You Know?

- "Sarcopenia limits muscle function with 25% of maximal force-generating capacity lost by age of 65 years and as much as 40% over a lifetime" (American College of Sports Medicine 2014).
- "Muscle mass declines annually approximately 1% to 2% after 50 years of age but muscle strength declines annually approximately 1% to 1.5% between 50 and 60 years of age and 3% after 60 years of age" (Legrand et al. 2013).
- An article by Naci et al. (2013) states that "although limited in quantity, existing randomised trial evidence on exercise interventions suggests that exercise and many drug interventions are often potentially similar in terms of their mortality benefits in the secondary prevention of coronary heart disease, rehabilitation after stroke, treatment of heart failure, and prevention of diabetes."
- "Muscle mass declines between 3% and 8% each decade after age 30. Muscle loss increases to 5% to 10% each decade after age 50" (Westcott 2012).
- "The human body is about 40% skeletal muscle and 10% smooth and cardiac muscle" (Hall 2011).
- "From 20 to 80 years of age, there is approximately a 30% reduction in muscle mass" (Evans 2010).
- Neumann (2010) states that "periods of reduced muscle activity lead to atrophy and usually marked reductions in strength, even in the first few weeks of inactivity. The loss in strength can occur early, up to 3% to 6% per day in the first week alone. After only 10 days of immobilization, healthy individuals can experience up to a 40% decrease of initial one-repetition maximum (1-RM)" (Appell 1990; Thom et al. 2001).

- "Healthy aged persons experience an approximate 10% per decade decline in peak strength after 60 years of age, with more rapid decline after 75 years of age" (Neumann 2010).
- Muscle mass is 70 percent to 75 percent water, whereas water in fat tissue can vary between 10 percent and 40 percent (Institute of Medicine of the National Academies 2005).
- "The loss of strength is primarily due to a loss of muscle tissue (muscle atrophy or sarcopenia) which has been calculated to amount to 1% or more per year after the age of 50. The annual decline in strength has been reported to be in the range of 1.4% to 5.4% per year" (Astrand et al. 2003).
- One pound of lean body mass (muscle) burns 14 calories per day and one pound of fat burns two calories per day (Heber 1999; Heber et al. 2001). As you increase your lean body mass, you burn more calories at rest and during activity.

References

American College of Sports Medicine. (2014). *ACSM's Resource Manual for Guidelines for Exercise Testing and Prescription*, 7th ed. Philadelphia, PA: Wolters Kluwer Lippincott Williams & Wilkins.

American College of Sports Medicine. (2014). *ACSM's Guidelines for Exercise Testing and Prescription*, 9th ed. Philadelphia, PA: Wolters Kluwer Lippincott Williams & Wilkins.

Appell HJ. (1990). Muscular atrophy following immobilisation. A review. *Sports Medicine* 10 (1): 42–58.

Astrand PO, Rodahl K, Dahl HA, et al. (2003). *Textbook of Work Physiology: The Physiological Bases of Exercise*, 4th ed. Champaign, IL: Human Kinetics.

Evans WJ. (2010). Skeletal muscle loss: Cachexia, sarcopenia, and inactivity. *American Journal of Clinical Nutrition* 91 (4): 1123S–1127S.

Hall JE. (2011). *Guyton and Hall Textbook of Medical Physiology*, 12th ed. Philadelphia, PA: Saunders Elsevier.

Halson SL. (2014). Monitoring training load to understand fatigue in athletes. *Sports Medicine* 44 (Supplement 2): 139–147.

Heber D. (1999). *The Resolution Diet: Keeping the Promise of Permanent Weight Loss*. Garden City Park, NY: Avery Publishing Group.

Heber D, and Bowerman S. (2001). *What Color is Your Diet? The 7 Colors of Health.* New York, NY: HarperCollins.

Hettinger T. (1961). *Physiology of Strength.* Springfield, IL: Charles C Thomas Publishers.

Hettinger T, and Muller EA. (1953). Muscle capacity and muscle training. *Arbeitsphysiologie* 15 (2): 111–126.

Institute of Medicine of the National Academies. (2005). *Water, Dietary Reference Intakes for Water, Sodium, Chloride, Potassium, and Sulfate.* Washington, DC: National Academy Press.

Kisner C, and Colby LA. (2012). *Therapeutic Exercise,* 6th ed. Philadelphia, PA: FA Davis.

Legrand D, Adriaensen W, Vaes B, et al. (2013). The relationship between grip strength and muscle mass (mm), inflammatory biomarkers and physical performance in community-dwelling very old persons. *Archives of Gerontology and Geriatrics* 57 (3): 345–351.

McGill SM. (2007). *Low Back Disorders,* 2nd ed. Champaign IL: Human Kinetics.

McGill SM. (2014). *Building the Ultimate Back: From Rehabilitation to Performance* (course manual). Los Angeles, CA, April 26–27.

McGill SM. (2014). *Ultimate Back Fitness and Performance,* 5th ed. Waterloo, Canada: Wabuno Publishers (Backfitpro Inc.). www.backfitpro.com.

McGill SM, Hughson RL, and Parks K. (2000). Lumbar erector spinae oxygenation during prolonged contractions: Implications for prolonged work. *Ergonomics* 43 (4): 486–493.

Naci H, and Ioannidis JP. (2013). Comparative effectiveness of exercise and drug interventions on mortality outcomes: Metaepidemiological study. *BMJ.* 347: f5577.

Neumann DA. (2010). *Kinesiology of the Musculoskeletal System: Foundations for Rehabilitation,* 2nd ed. St. Louis: Mosby Elsevier.

Pahor M, Guralnik JM, Ambrosius WT, et al. (2014). Effect of structured physical activity on prevention of major mobility disability in older adults: The life study randomized clinical trial. *JAMA* 311 (23): 2387–2396.

Thom JM, Thompson MW, Ruell PA, et al. (2001). Effect of 10-day cast immobilization on sarcoplasmic reticulum calcium regulation in humans. *Acta Physiologica Scandinavica* 172 (2): 141–147.

Venes D. (Ed.) (2013). *Taber's Cyclopedic Medical Dictionary,* 22nd ed. Philadelphia, PA: FA Davis.

Verkhoshansky Y, and Siff M. (2009). *Supertraining,* 6th ed. Rome, Italy: Verkhoshansky. www.verkhoshansky.com.

Verkhoshansky Y, and Verkhoshansky N. (2011). *Special Strength Training Manual for Coaches*. Rome Italy: Verkhoshansky SSTM. www.verkhoshansky.com.

Westcott WL. (2012). Resistance training is medicine: effects of strength training on health. *Current Sports Medicine Reports* 11 (4): 209–216.

PART 6
Improving Brain Health

Cognition can be defined as thinking skills, language use, perception, calculation, awareness, memory, reasoning, judgment, learning, intellect, social skills, and imagination (Venes 2013). Cognitive function (or "executive function") impairments in individuals can lead to difficulties with activities of daily living, such as dressing, eating, bathing, toileting, and walking. Additionally, a decline of cognitive function can result in reduced quality of life and problems with social engagement, driving skills, work-related tasks, money management, shopping, and operating communication devices (Jobe et al. 2001).

The following areas show promise in enhancing cognitive function, or slowing its decline, and also in maintaining mental stability:

Acupressure Routine for Alertness
See an acupuncturist for detailed instructions. Try stimulating the following acupressure points for three minutes each to help increase your alertness before a test (Harris et al. 2005):

- Si Shen Chong point—lightly tap the top of the head
- LI 4 point—massage the web space between the thumb and index finger
- St 36 point—massage the point located about four finger widths down from the bottom of your knee cap, on the outer boundary of your shin bone
- K 1 point—massage the front portion of the bottom of your foot between the web space of the second and third toe
- UB 10 point—massage the depression at the outer border of the back of your neck within the hairline

Aerobic Training

Engaging in any aerobic exercise and physical activity, such as walking or jogging, elevates heart health but can also keep your brain healthy (Alves et al. 2014; Baker et al. 2010; Buck et al. 2008; Carvalho et al. 2014; Chapman et al. 2014; Chang et al. 2015; Fabel et al. 2008; Hillman et al. 2003, 2009; Li et al. 2014; Nanda et al. 2013; Pontifex et al. 2009; ten Brinke 2015; Voss et al. 2010; Winter et al. 2007; Wu et al. 2011; Zhao et al. 2014; Zhu et al. 2014). Some studies have shown certain aspects of cognition in children can improve with exercise (Drollette et al. 2014; Fedewa et al. 2011; Kirkendall 1986; Lees et al. 2013; Tomporowski et al. 2008).

A study by Gauthier et al. (2015) indicates that "cognitive status in aging is linked to vascular health, and that preservation of vessel elasticity may be one of the key mechanisms by which physical exercise helps to alleviate cognitive aging." These findings are in line with other research, which studied older women (Brown et al. 2010). Moreover, a study by Guiney et al. (2015) shows that healthy young adults, ages 18 to 30, who engage in physical activity might improve their cognitive function. An article by Phillips et al. (2015) states that "In summary, the data presented here suggests that moderate physical activity—a target that is practical, well tolerated, and likely to optimize exercise adherence—can be used to improve cognitive function and reduce the slope of cognitive decline in people with dementia of the Alzheimer disease type."

So walk, bike, hike, swim, or do some other aerobic activity at least three to five times per week.

Dancing

Tango dancing and mindfulness meditation can be effective complementary adjuncts for the treatment of depression as a part of stress-management programs (Pinniger et al. 2012).

Diet and Medical Conditions

Be aware of your diet and how it can impact certain medical conditions. For example, a study by Lichtwark et al. (2014) indicates that "in newly diagnosed coeliac disease [also spelled "celiac," an immunologic intolerance to dietary wheat products, especially gluten and gliadin], cognitive performance improves with adherence to the gluten-free diet in parallel to mucosal healing. Suboptimal levels of cognition in untreated coeliac disease may affect the performance of everyday tasks" (Venes 2013). See your physician and discuss any concerns you may have regarding your sensitivity to gluten or any other food.

Eat Quality Foods

Quality foods can help enhance your brain function. The following are studies showing the link between food and cognitive function:

- Even following a short-term (10 days in this study) Mediterranean-style diet has the potential to enhance certain aspects of mood, cognition, and cardiovascular function in young healthy adults (Lee et al. 2015).
- A study by Smyth et al. (2015) indicates that a "higher diet quality was associated with a reduced risk of cognitive decline. Improved diet quality represents an important potential target for reducing the global burden of cognitive decline."
- A study by Valls-Pedret et al. (2015) indicates that "In an older population [average age in the study was 66.9 years], a Mediterranean diet supplemented with olive oil or nuts is associated with improved cognitive function."

Folic Acid

A study by Agnew-Blais et al. (2015) indicates that "folate intake below the Recommended Daily Allowance may increase risk for MCI [mild cognitive impairment]/probable dementia in later life."

Food for Thought

An article by Rampersaud et al. (2005) indicates "that breakfast consumption may improve cognitive function related to memory, test grades, and school attendance" in children and adolescents. Also, a balanced diet with sufficient calories and nutrients are needed to prevent nutritional imbalances. The following foods and nutrients have been shown to positively affect cognitive function:

- *Blueberries*—A study by Krikorian et al. (2010) indicates that "moderate-term blueberry supplementation can confer neurocognitive benefit."
- *Fish and omega-3 oils*—A study by Barberger-Gateau et al. (2007) indicates that "frequent consumption of fruits and vegetables, fish, and omega-3 rich oils may decrease the risk of dementia and Alzheimer's disease."
- *Green leafy vegetables*—A study by Kang et al. (2005) indicates that "women consuming the most green leafy vegetables also experienced slower [cognitive] decline than women consuming the least amount."
- *Plants/Extracts*—Plants and their extracts, such as saffron, ginseng, sage, lemon balm, and Ginkgo biloba, have produced some promising clinical data for

individuals with dementia pathologies such as Alzheimer's disease (Howes et al. 2011).

- *Pomegranate juice*—A study by Bookheimer et al. (2013) indicates that "results suggest a role for pomegranate juice in augmenting memory function through task-related increases in functional brain activity."
- *Turmeric*—An article by Ng et al. (2006) indicates that "curcumin, from the curry spice turmeric, has been shown to possess potent antioxidant and anti-inflammatory properties and to reduce beta-amyloid and plaque burden in experimental studies" and also that "those who consumed curry 'occasionally' and 'often or very often' had significantly better MMSE [mini-mental state examination] scores than did subjects who 'never or rarely' consumed curry."
- *Water*—Water helps prevent dehydration, which may impair mood and cognitive performance (Cheuvront et al. 2014; Masento et al. 2014).

Gut and Brain Health

Are you in a bad mood? Are you depressed or anxious? Are you having a hard time focusing or concentrating? Do you have uncontrolled anger? Your gut could be the blame. More than likely, one of the next big areas in medicine is going to focus on the interactions between the gastrointestinal system and the brain and how this can affect our sense of well-being. Therefore, exploring all options to improve health is a part of good medical practice and wellness.

The body's largest immune organ is the gastrointestinal tract. It has nearly 100 trillion bacteria, or about one kilogram of bacteria in the adult gut which are essential for health (Dinan et al. 2015; Foster et al. 2013; Severance et al. 2015). Microorganisms make up about one to three percent of our body mass (that's two to six pounds of bacteria in a 200-pound adult) (Human Microbiome Project 2015).

According to the Human Microbiome Project website (http://hmpdacc.org), microorganisms in the human body "produce some vitamins that we do not have the genes to make, break down our food to extract nutrients we need to survive, teach our immune systems how to recognize dangerous invaders and even produce helpful anti-inflammatory compounds that fight off other disease-causing microbes."

Research says...

- McKean et al. (2016) state that "probiotic consumption may have a positive effect on psychological symptoms of depression, anxiety, and perceived stress in healthy human volunteers."

- Huang et al. (2016) concluded that "probiotics were associated with a significant reduction in depression."
- Keightley et al. (2015) state that "Psychological treatments are known to improve functional gastrointestinal disorders, the next wave of research may involve preventative microbiological gut based treatments for primary psychological presentations, both to treat the presenting complaint and inoculate against later functional gastrointestinal disorders."
- Severance et al. (2015) state that "With accumulating evidence supporting newly discovered gut-brain physiological pathways, treatments to ameliorate brain symptoms of schizophrenia should be supplemented with therapies to correct gastrointestinal dysfunction."

Improving Gut and Brain Function

The following are some tips to help improve digestion and maintain a healthy gastrointestinal system:

- Follow medical treatment guidelines for conditions such as irritable bowel syndrome, Celiac disease, and Crohn disease.
- Get regular dental checkups. Also, brush and floss your teeth and massage your gums daily to keep your mouth healthy to prevent gastrointestinal illness.
- Identify and control food allergens, intolerances, and sensitivities (Daulatzai 2015; Nemani et al. 2015) and malabsorption problems (such as lactose or fructose).
- Control your stress.
- Don't smoke (Fujiwara et al. 2011).
- Limit alcohol consumption (Swanson et al. 2010).
- Limit caffeine consumption (Heizer et al. 2009).
- Get enough sleep to help prevent stress and ensure full recovery (Chen et al. 2011).
- Exercise daily to help digestion and prevent constipation (Klare et al. 2015).
- Eat slowly to prevent not only overeating, but to also aid in proper digestion.
- Avoid large meals (Heizer et al. 2009)
- Practice mindfulness meditation.
- Eat a varied and balanced diet to avoid nutritional deficiencies.
- Wash your hands thoroughly before eating to prevent gastrointestinal illness (Aiello et al. 2008).

- Give your mouth a quick rinse with water before you eat (especially in the morning after you awaken) to avoid swallowing unnecessary bacteria which has built up in your mouth overnight. Even though more research is needed in this area before additional guidelines may be provided, it is a simple habit which causes no harm.
- Consider storing your floss, toothbrush, and gum massager outside of your bathroom to avoid cross contamination from your toilet (American Society for Microbiology 2015).
- Consider seeing a health care practitioner specializing in aromatherapy massage for relief of constipation, indigestion, nausea, or loss of appetite using essential oils.
- Consider seeing an acupuncturist for acupuncture and acupressure techniques for gastrointestinal health (Cross 2001).
- Include prebiotics and probiotics into your diet (Scott et al. 2015).
  - **Prebiotics** - A nutrient that stimulates the growth or health of bacteria living in the large intestine (Venes 2013). Prebiotics occur naturally in foods such as fruits, vegetables, barley, flax, legumes, and oats (Gensler 2008). Prebiotics from foods can reduce the prevalence and duration of infectious and antibiotic-associated diarrhea, reduce the inflammation and symptoms of inflammatory bowel disease, protect against colon cancer, enhance the bioavailability and uptake of minerals (such as calcium, magnesium, and possibly iron), lower some risk for cardiovascular disease, and promote weight loss and prevent obesity (Slavin 2013).
  - **Probiotics** - Having favorable or health-promoting effect on living cells and tissues (Venes 2013). Probiotics occur naturally in foods such as yogurt, kefir, miso, and tempeh (Gensler 2008). Also, Kombucha tea and other cultured vegetables contain probiotics. Probiotics from foods or supplements can prevent hypercholesterolemia (excessive amount of cholesterol in the blood), upper respiratory tract infections, bacterial vaginosis (vaginal infection), and antibiotic-associated diarrhea, help manage constipation, and reduce recurrent urinary tract infections and irritable bowel syndrome symptoms (Taibi et al. 2014).

Did You Know?

- "It takes about 3 to 4 weeks for a complete turnover of all gut cells throughout the digestive tract" (Goodman et al. 2015).

- "Because two-thirds of all immune system function and 90% of serotonin function take place in the gut, healing the gut can assist in bringing both of these functions back into balance. Serotonin is needed to produce melatonin, which is an essential component for good, restful sleep; the proper amount of circulating and functioning serotonin is also needed to stabilize mood" (Goodman et al. 2015).

Meditation

A study by Wells et al. (2013) indicates that "Mindfulness-Based Stress Reduction (MBSR) may have a positive impact on the regions of the brain most related to mild cognitive impairment and Alzheimer's disease." Another article indicates mindfulness meditation reduces anxiety (Zeidan et al. 2014).

Memory Fitness Program

Look into enrolling in a memory fitness program at your local college, university, or community center. A study by Miller et al. (2012) indicates that, "a 6-week healthy lifestyle program can improve both encoding and recalling of new verbal information, as well as self-perception of memory ability in older adults residing in continuing care retirement communities." Another study by Small et al. (2006) states that "a short-term healthy lifestyle program combining mental and physical exercise, stress reduction, and healthy diet was associated with significant effects on cognitive function and brain metabolism."

Minimize Pollution

A study by Wilker et al. (2015) suggests that "Air pollution is associated with insidious effects on structural brain aging even in dementia and stroke-free persons."

Net-Step Exercise

A study by Kitazawa et al. (2015) created a simple recreational stepping program using a Fumanet to maintain cognitive health and gait function. The name "Fumanet Exercise" originates from the words *fumanai* (which means "to avoid stepping on something" in Japanese) and "net exercise" (Sompo Japan Research Institute 2010). Also, view the video at http://links.lww.com/JGPT/A4 for the basics of how to perform the stepping program.

Night and Day

Get adequate rest, relaxation, and sleep. A study by Yoo et al. (2007) indicates that "results demonstrate that an absence of prior sleep substantially compromises the neural and behavioral capacity for committing new experiences to memory. It therefore appears that sleep before learning is critical in preparing the human brain for next-day memory formation—a worrying finding considering society's increasing erosion of sleep time." On the flip side, get enough natural bright light every day to increase the brain's serotonin levels needed to enhance mood and vitality (Brawley 2009).

No Smoking and Limited Alcohol

A study by Hagger-Johnson et al. (2013) indicates that "smokers who drank alcohol heavily had a 36% faster cognitive decline, equivalent to an age-effect of 2 extra years over 10-year follow-up, compared with individuals who were non-smoking moderate drinkers." Another study by Sabia et al. (2014) indicates that "excessive alcohol consumption in men was associated with faster cognitive decline compared with light to moderate alcohol consumption" (Kabai 2014).

Rocking Chair

Rocking in a rocking chair for 30 minutes might increase blood flow to the brain (Pierce et al. 2009).

Soothing Music

Listening to music leads to positive changes in a person's emotional state and decreases the severity of behavioral disorders (Narme et al. 2013). Music also appears to reduce depression in elderly individuals (Chu et al. 2013).

Stable Blood Glucose Levels

Keep your blood sugar levels stable throughout your life. The following are studies showing the link between blood glucose and cognitive function:

- Weinstein et al. (2015) indicates that "hyperglycemia is associated with subtle brain injury and impaired attention and memory even in young adults, indicating that brain injury is an early manifestation of impaired glucose metabolism."
- Roberts et al. (2014) indicates that "Midlife onset of diabetes may affect late-life cognition through loss of brain volume."
- Young et al. (2014) indicates that "The ability to control the levels of blood glucose was related to mood and cognition."
- Crane et al. (2013) indicates that "higher glucose levels may be a risk factor for dementia, even among persons without diabetes."

Stable Blood Pressure

Reducing your blood pressure can affect cognitive function in a positive way. One study (Roberts et al. 2014) indicates that "midlife hypertension may affect executive function through ischemic pathology." An article by Nagai et al. (2010) concludes that "brain matter damage caused by long-standing hypertensive status is associated with cognitive impairment. Accordingly, strict blood pressure control including during sleep may have a neuroprotective effect on the brain, and thereby prevent the incidence of dementia."

Steroid Use for Muscle Building

Androgenic-anabolic steroid use among regular gym users impairs memory (Heffernan et al. 2015).

Strength Training

Many studies show that engaging in strength training exercises (using resistance) has positive effects on cognitive function (Altug 2014; Brown et al. 2009; Cancela Carral et al. 2007; Cassilhas et al. 2007; Chang et al. 2009, 2012, 2014; Forte et al. 2013; Fragala et al. 2014; Kimura et al. 2010; Komulainen et al. 2010; Liu-Ambrose et al. 2008, 2010, 2012; Ozkaya et al. 2005; Perrig-Chiello et al. 1998; Tsutsumi et al. 1997).

Research says...

- A study by Fiatarone et al. (2014) indicates that "resistance training significantly improved global cognitive function, with maintenance of executive and global benefits over 18 months" in men and women ages 55 or above with mild cognitive impairment.
- A study by Fragala et al. (2014) indicates that "resistance exercise training may be an effective means to preserve or improve spatial awareness and reaction with aging" in adults over 60 years old.
- A study by Liu-Ambrose et al. (2010) indicates that "twelve months of once-weekly or twice-weekly resistance training benefited the executive cognitive function of selective attention and conflict resolution among senior women [ages 65 to 75]."

So why wait? Start doing some resistance training at least twice a week. Use equipment such as hand and ankle weights, or do exercises like push-ups that use the weight of your own body as resistance.

Stress Relief

Reduce daily stress levels (Lupien et al. 2005). A study indicates that controlling "anxiety symptoms may help delay memory decline in otherwise healthy older adults" (Pietrzak et al. 2014).

Test Taking Strategies

Should you be physically active (such as walking, walking in place, or doing simple calisthenics) just before a major test or other mentally difficult task (such as a physician before surgery, a speaker before a lecture, or an airline pilot just before taking off or landing)? Even though some researchers suggest that the results of cognitive improvement with exercise should be interpreted cautiously based on current studies, why wait or take a chance that something as simple as some exercise before a test or a mentally challenging task can give you an advantage? How much would school and work performance improve if every student and worker was allowed multiple mini-exercise breaks throughout the day, especially before a mentally challenging task?

Perhaps the reason some people get good ideas during a shower or long walk is due to increased blood flow to the brain. Or is it due to the relaxation? Either way, engaging in low-key activities is good for you. Why not get up and move around or go for a 10- to 30-minute walk, and see what happens? Maybe even make your next meeting a "walking meeting" with your client or staff. You would be in good company since many great thinkers, like Aristotle, Ludwig van Beethoven, Charles Darwin, Charles Dickens, Albert Einstein, Steve Jobs, and Friedrich Nietzsche, used walking as a part of their thinking and creative process.

Sample Test Taking Routine

As with any athletic program, there is a trial-and-error period to find the precise combination of what will work on test day. Try some or all of the following tips before your next test:

- The most important part is to study your materials well in advance of a test. No all-nighters!
- Get enough sleep the previous night.
- Eat a healthful breakfast before the test.
- Get some natural outdoor sunlight in the morning before the test.
- Perform light exercises, such as walking or calisthenics before the test, for 10 to 30 minutes to invigorate your body and increase blood flow to your brain.

- Use diaphragmatic breathing to relax before the test. Just before your test (or any intense mental task), close your eyes to relax, and breathe diaphragmatically 10 times in a slow and controlled manner.
- To reduce test anxiety before the test, consider trying the Emotional Freedom Technique (Benor et al. 2009).
- Try smelling a <u>little</u> rosemary oil (Diego et al. 1998) or peppermint oil (Moss et al. 2008) before a test to help increase your alertness. Just remember, peppermint to "pep" you up.

Vitamin D

The following studies are related to vitamin D and cognition, indicating that having your vitamin D level checked is another good reason to get annual medical checkups:

- Afzal et al. (2014) "observed an association of reduced plasma 25(OH)D with increased risk of the combined end point of Alzheimer's disease and vascular dementia in this prospective cohort study of the general population."
- Pettersen et al. (2014) indicates that "vitamin D3 insufficiency and seasonal declines ≥ [greater than or equal to] 15 nmol/L were associated with inferior working memory/executive functioning."
- Llewellyn et al. (2010) indicates that "low levels of vitamin D were associated with substantial cognitive decline in the elderly population studied over a six-year period."
- Seamans et al. (2010) indicates that "low vitamin D status was associated with a reduced capacity for SWM (spatial working memory), particularly in women" in several European countries.

Yoga or Tai Chi

Studies indicate that yoga may lead to improvements in cognitive function (Gothe et al. 2014; Hariprasad et al. 2013). Another study indicates that "mind-body exercise with integrated cognitive and motor coordination may help with the preservation of global ability in elders at risk of cognitive decline" (Lam et al. 2012).

Play Some Mind Games

A study by Miller (2013) indicates that "participating in a computerized brain exercise program over 6 months improves cognitive abilities in older adults." Try the following games to stimulate your brain cells:

- Bridge, www.bridgebase.com
- Cards, www.solitaire-cardgame.com
- Chess, www.chess.com
- Crossword puzzles, www.boatloadpuzzles.com
- Dakim BrainFitness, www.dakim.com
- Fit Brains, www.fitbrains.com
- Lumosity, www.lumosity.com
- Sudoku, www.247sudoku.com

Stay Engaged in Life

Be socially interactive by joining clubs, volunteering, or teaching (Ybarra et al. 2008). Experience something beyond your normal activities. Go to a museum, opera, theater, or sporting event. Try something new and novel in your life, such as the following:

- Art—take drawing, painting, or sculpting classes
- Community involvement—volunteer, coach, or organize in your community
- Continued education—take a class at a community college (Hatch et al. 2007)
- Cooking—learn to cook and try new recipes
- Dance—take ballroom, hip-hop, or tango classes
- Language—take French or Chinese classes (Alladi et al. 2013; Craik et al. 2010)
- Math—do occasional simple arithmetic in your head
- Music—take lessons in flute, piano, or guitar
- Poetry—uncover hidden meanings or pen your own poems
- Reading—read newspapers, books, or magazines
- Writing—try journaling, writing prose, or work on your best-selling novel!

Brain Fitness Coordination Exercise Routine

Simple coordination exercises improve cognitive function in men and women ages 66 to 90 (Kwok et al. 2011). Try the following modified movement circuit while sitting in a chair:

- Keep your eyes focused ahead while turning your head slowly to the right and left. Now keep your eyes focused ahead while moving your head slowly up and down.

- Touch your nose, alternating right and left index fingers. Now touch your ears, again alternating right and left index fingers.
- Turn the palms of both hands alternately to face up and down with elbows bent to 90 degrees.
- Touch your right or left shoulder, hip, or knee depending on the verbal commands of a training partner. Slowly increase the speed of the verbal commands. Try it with your eyes closed.
- Draw patterns (such as a circle, triangle, square, or rectangle) or letters of the alphabet in the air in front of your body with your right or left hand. Try this, too, with your eyes closed.
- Slide the heel of your right leg up along your left shin. Alternate legs. Again, try it with your closed eyes.

Did You Know?

- The metabolism of the brain accounts for about 15 percent of the total metabolism in the body under resting but awake conditions. The mass of the brain is only 2 percent of total body mass (Hall 2011).
- "Collectively, the brain, liver, heart, and kidneys account for approximately 60% to 70% of resting energy expenditure in adults, whereas their combined weight is less than 6% of total body weight. Skeletal muscle comprises 40% to 50% of total body weight and accounts for only 20% to 30% of resting energy expenditure" (Javed et al. 2010).

References

Afzal S, Bojesen SE, and Nordestgaard BG. (2014). Reduced 25-hydroxyvitamin D and risk of Alzheimer's disease and vascular dementia. *Alzheimer's & Dementia* 10 (3): 296–302.

Agnew-Blais JC, Wassertheil-Smoller S, Kang JH, et al. (2015). Folate, vitamin B-6, and vitamin B-12 intake and mild cognitive impairment and probable dementia in the Women's Health Initiative Memory Study. *Journal of the Academy of Nutrition and Dietetics* 115 (2): 231–241.

Aiello AE, Coulborn RM, Perez V, et al. (2008). Effect of hand hygiene on infectious disease risk in the community setting: A meta-analysis. *American Journal of Public Health* 98 (8): 1372–1381.

Alladi S, Bak TH, Duggirala V, et al. (2013). Bilingualism delays age at onset of dementia, independent of education and immigration status. *Neurology* 81 (22): 1938–1944.

Altug Z. (2016). Constipation and low back pain in an athlete: A case report. *Orthopaedic Physical Therapy Practice*. 28 (3): 188-192.

Altug Z. (2014). Resistance exercise to improve cognitive function. *Strength and Conditioning Journal* 36 (6): 46–50.

Alves CR, Tessaro VH, Teixeira LA, et al. (2014). Influence of acute high-intensity aerobic interval exercise bout on selective attention and short-term memory tasks. *Perceptual and Motor Skills* 118 (1): 63–72.

American Society for Microbiology. (2015). *Toothbrush contamination in communal bathrooms*. American Society for Microbiology. Retrieved on July 11, 2015 from www.asm.org/index.php/press-releases/93536-toothbrush-contamination-in-communal-bathrooms

Baker LD, Frank LL, Foster-Schubert K, et al. (2010). Aerobic exercise improves cognition for older adults with glucose intolerance, a risk factor for Alzheimer's disease. *Journal of Alzheimer's Disease* 22 (2): 569–579.

Barberger-Gateau P, Raffaitin C, Letenneur L, et al. (2007). Dietary patterns and risk of dementia: The Three-City cohort study. *Neurology* 69 (20): 1921–1930.

Barral JP. (2007). *Visceral Manipulation II*, revised edition. Seattle, WA: Eastland Press.

Barral JP, and Mercier P. (2005). *Visceral Manipulation*, revised edition. Seattle, WA: Eastland Press.

Benor DJ., Ledger K, Toussaint L, et al. (2009). Pilot study of emotional freedom techniques, wholistic hybrid derived from eye movement desensitization and reprocessing and emotional freedom technique, and cognitive behavioral therapy for treatment of test anxiety in university students. *Explore (NY)* 5 (6): 338–340.

Bookheimer SY, Renner BA, Ekstrom A, et al. (2013). Pomegranate juice augments memory and FMRI activity in middle-aged and older adults with mild memory complaints. *Evidence-Based Complementary and Alternative Medicine* 946298.

Brawley EC. (2009). Enriching light design. *NeuroRehabilitation* 25 (3): 189–199.

Bredesen DE. (2014). Reversal of cognitive decline: A novel therapeutic program. *Aging (Albany NY)* 6 (9): 707–717.

Brown AD, McMorris CA, Longman RS, et al. (2010). Effects of cardiorespiratory fitness and cerebral blood flow on cognitive outcomes in older women. *Neurobiology of Aging.* 31 (12): 2047–2057.

Brown AK, Liu-Ambrose T, Tate R, et al. (2009). The effect of group-based exercise on cognitive performance and mood in seniors residing in intermediate care and self-care retirement facilities: A randomised controlled trial. *British Journal of Sports Medicine* 43 (8): 608–614.

Buck SM, Hillman CH, and Castelli DM. (2008). The relation of aerobic fitness to Stroop task performance in preadolescent children. *Medicine and Science in Sports and Exercise* 40 (1): 166–172.

Cancela Carral JM, and Ayan Perez C. (2007). Effects of high-intensity combined training on women over 65. *Gerontology* 53 (6): 340–346.

Carpenter S. (2012). That gut feeling. *Monitor on Psychology* 43 (8): 50.

Carvalho A, Rea IM, Parimon T, et al. (2014). Physical activity and cognitive function in individuals over 60 years of age: A systematic review. *Clinical Interventions in Aging.* 9: 661–682.

Cassilhas RC, Viana VA, Grassmann V, et al. (2007). The impact of resistance exercise on the cognitive function of the elderly. *Medicine and Science in Sports and Exercise* 39 (8): 1401–1407.

Chang YK, Chu CH, Wang CC et al. (2015). Dose–response relation between exercise duration and cognition. *Medicine & Science in Sports & Exercise* 47 (1): 159–165.

Chang YK, and Etnier JL. (2009). Effects of an acute bout of localized resistance exercise on cognitive performance in middle-aged adults: A randomized controlled trial study. *Psychology of Sport and Exercise* 10 (1): 19–24.

Chang YK, Ku PW, Tomporowski PD, et al. (2012). Effects of acute resistance exercise on late-middle-age adults' goal planning. *Medicine and Science in Sports and Exercise* 44 (9): 1773–1779.

Chang YK, Tsai CL, Huang CC, et al. (2014). Effects of acute resistance exercise on cognition in late middle-aged adults: General or specific cognitive improvement? *Journal of Science and Medicine in Sport* 17 (1): 51–55.

Chen CL, Liu TT, Yi CH, et al. (2011). Evidence for altered anorectal function in irritable bowel syndrome patients with sleep disturbance. *Digestion* 84 (3): 247–251.

Chapman SB, Aslan S, Spence JS, et al. (2013). Shorter term aerobic exercise improves brain, cognition, and cardiovascular fitness in aging. *Frontiers in Aging Neuroscience* 5: 75.

Chapman SB, Aslan S, Spence JS, et al. (2015). Neural mechanisms of brain plasticity with complex cognitive training in healthy seniors. *Cerebral Cortex* 25 (2): 396–405.

Cheuvront SN, and Kenefick RW. (2014). Dehydration: Physiology, assessment, and performance effects. *Comprehensive Physiology* 4 (1): 257–285.

Chodzko-Zajko O, Kramer A, and Poon L. (2009). *Enhancing Cognitive Functioning and Brain Plasticity* (Volume 3). Champaign, IL: Human Kinetics.

Chu H, Yang CY, Lin Y, et al. (2013). The Impact of group music therapy on depression and cognition in elderly persons with dementia: A randomized controlled study. *Biological Research for Nursing* 16 (2): 209–217.

Craik FI, Bialystok E, and Freedman M. (2010). Delaying the onset of Alzheimer disease: Bilingualism as a form of cognitive reserve. *Neurology* 75 (19): 1726–1729.

Crane PK, Walker R, Hubbard RA, et al. (2013). Glucose levels and risk of dementia. *New England Journal of Medicine* 369 (6): 540–548.

Cross JR. (2001). Acupressure & Reflextherapy in the Treatment of Medical Conditions. London, England: Butterworth-Heinemann.

Daulatzai MA. (2015). Non-celiac gluten sensitivity triggers gut dysbiosis, neuroinflammation, gut-brain axis dysfunction, and vulnerability for dementia. *CNS & Neurological Disorders Drug Targets* 14 (1): 110–131.

Diego MA, Jones NA, Field T, et al. (1998). Aromatherapy positively affects mood, EEG patterns of alertness and math computations. *International Journal of Neuroscience* 96 (3-4): 217–224.

Di Lazzaro V, Capone F, Cammarota G, et al. (2014). Dramatic improvement of Parkinsonian symptoms after gluten-free diet introduction in a patient with silent celiac disease. *Journal of Neurology*, 261 (2): 443–445.

Dinan TG, Stilling RM, Stanton C, et al. (2015). Collective unconscious: How gut microbes shape human behavior. *Journal of Psychiatric Research* 63: 1–9.

Drollette ES, Scudder MR, Raine LB, et al. (2014). Acute exercise facilitates brain function and cognition in children who need it most: An ERP study of individual differences in inhibitory control capacity. *Developmental Cognitive Neuroscience* 7: 53–64.

Fabel K, and Kempermann G. (2008). Physical activity and the regulation of neurogenesis in the adult and aging brain. *NeuroMolecular Medicine* 10 (2): 59–66.

Fedewa AL, and Ahn S. (2011). The effects of physical activity and physical fitness on children's achievement and cognitive outcomes: A meta-analysis. *Research Quarterly for Exercise and Sport* 82 (3): 521–535.

Fernandez A, Goldberg E, and Michelon P. (2013). *The SharpBrains Guide to Brain Fitness.* San Francisco, CA: SharpBrain Inc. http://sharpbrains.com.

Fiatarone Singh MA, Gates N, Saigal N, et al. (2014). The study of mental and resistance training (SMART) study-resistance training and/or cognitive training in mild cognitive impairment: A randomized, double-blind, double-sham controlled trial. *Journal of the American Medical Directors Association* 15 (12): 873–880.

Forte R, Boreham CA, Leite JC, et al. (2013). Enhancing cognitive functioning in the elderly: Multicomponent vs resistance training. *Clinical Interventions in Aging* 8: 19–27.

Foster JA, and McVey Neufeld KA. (2013). Gut-brain axis: How the microbiome influences anxiety and depression. *Trends in Neurosciences* 36 (5): 305–312.

Fragala MS, Beyer KS, Jajtner AR, et al. (2014). Resistance exercise may improve spatial awareness and visual reaction in older adults. *Journal of Strength and Conditioning Research* 28 (8): 2079–2087.

Fujiwara Y, Kubo M, and Kohata Y. (2011). Cigarette smoking and its association with overlapping gastroesophageal reflux disease, functional dyspepsia, or irritable bowel syndrome. *Internal Medicine (Tokyo, Japan)* 50 (21): 2443–2447.

Gauthier CJ, Lefort M, Mekary S, et al. (2015). Hearts and minds: Linking vascular rigidity and aerobic fitness with cognitive aging. *Neurobiology of Aging* 36 (1): 304–314.

Gensler TO. (2008). Probiotic and Prebiotic Recipes for Health: 100 Recipes That Battle Colitis, Candidiasis, Food Allergies, and Other Digestive Disorders. Beverly, MA: Fair Wind Press.

Goodman CC, and Fuller KS. (2015). *Pathology: Implications for the Physical Therapist,* 4rd ed. St. Louis, MO: Elsevier Saunders.

Gothe NP, Kramer AF, and McAuley E. (2014). The effects of an 8-week hatha yoga intervention on executive function in older adults. *Journals of Gerontology. Series A, Biological Sciences and Medical Sciences* 69 (9): 1109–1116.

Guiney H, Lucas SJ, Cotter JD, et al. (2015). Evidence cerebral blood-flow regulation mediates exercise-cognition links in healthy young adults. *Neuropsychology* 29 (1): 1–9.

Hagger-Johnson G, Sabia S, Brunner EJ, et al. (2013). Combined impact of smoking and heavy alcohol use on cognitive decline in early old age: Whitehall II prospective cohort study. *British Journal of Psychiatry* 203 (2): 120–125.

Hall JE. (2011). *Guyton and Hall Textbook of Medical Physiology*, 12th ed. Philadelphia, PA: Saunders Elsevier.

Hariprasad VR, Koparde V, Sivakumar PT, et al. (2013). Randomized clinical trial of yoga-based intervention in residents from elderly homes: Effects on cognitive function. *Indian Journal Psychiatry* 55 (Supplement 3): S357–363.

Harris RE, Jeter J, Chan P, et al. (2005). Using acupressure to modify alertness in the classroom: A single-blinded, randomized, cross-over trial. *Journal of Alternative and Complementary Medicine* 11 (4): 673–679.

Hatch SL, Feinstein L, Link BG, et al. (2007). The continuing benefits of education: Adult education and midlife cognitive ability in the British 1946 birth cohort. *Journals of Gerontology. Series B, Psychological Sciences and Social Sciences* 62 (6): S404–414.

Heffernan TM, Battersby L, Bishop P, et al. (2015). Everyday memory deficits associated with anabolic-androgenic steroid use in regular gymnasium users. *The Open Psychiatry Journal* 9: 1–6.

Heizer WD, Southern S, and McGovern, S. (2009). The role of diet in symptoms of irritable bowel syndrome in adults: A narrative review. *Journal of the American Dietetic Association* 109 (7): 1204–1214.

Hillman CH, Pontifex MB, Raine LB, et al. (2009). The effect of acute treadmill walking on cognitive control and academic achievement in preadolescent children. *Neuroscience* 159 (3): 1044–1054.

Hillman CH, Snook EM, and Jerome GJ. (2003). Acute cardiovascular exercise and executive control function. *International Journal of Psychophysiology* 48 (3): 307–314.

Howes MJ, and Perry E. (2011). The role of phytochemicals in the treatment and prevention of dementia. *Drugs & Aging* 28 (6): 439–468.

Huang R, Wang, K, Hu J. (2016). Effect of probiotics on depression: A systematic review and meta-analysis of randomized controlled trials. *Nutrients* 8 (8).

Hulsken S, Martin A, Mohajeri MH, et al. (2013). Food-derived serotonergic modulators: Effects on mood and cognition. *Nutrition Research Reviews* 26 (2): 223–234.

Human Microbiome Project. (2015). *About the Human Microbiome Project.* Bethesda, MD: National Institutes of Health. Retrieved on July 11, 2015 from http://hmp-dacc.org/overview/about.php.

Javed F, He Q, Davidson LE, et al. (2010). Brain and high metabolic rate organ mass: Contributions to resting energy expenditure beyond fat-free mass. *American Journal of Clinical Nutrition* 91 (4): 907–912.

Jobe JB, Smith DM, Ball K, et al. (2001). ACTIVE: a cognitive intervention trial to promote independence in older adults. *Controlled Clinical Trials* 22 (4): 453–479.

Kabai P. (2014). Alcohol consumption and cognitive decline in early old age. *Neurology* 83 (5): 476.

Kang JH, Ascherio A, and Grodstein F. (2005). Fruit and vegetable consumption and cognitive decline in aging women. *Annals of Neurology* 57 (5): 713–720.

Keightley PC, Koloski NA, and Talley NJ. (2015). Pathways in gut-brain communication: Evidence for distinct gut-to-brain and brain-to-gut syndromes. *Australian and New Zealand Journal of Psychiatry* 49 (3): 207–214.

Kimura K, Obuchi S, Arai T, et al. (2010). The influence of short-term strength training on health-related quality of life and executive cognitive function. *Journal of Physiological Anthropology* 29 (3): 95–101.

Kirkendall DR. (1986). Effects of physical activity on intellectual development and academic performance. In: Lee M, Eckert HM, and Stull GA. (Eds.). *Effects of Physical Activity on Children: A Special Tribute to Mabel Lee.* Champaign, IL: Human Kinetics.

Kitazawa K, Showa S, Hiraoka A, et al. (2015). Effect of a dual-task net-step exercise on cognitive and gait function in older adults. *Journal of Geriatric Physical Therapy* 38 (3): 133–140.

Klare P, Nigg J, Nold J, et al. (2015). The impact of a ten-week physical exercise program on health-related quality of life in patients with inflammatory bowel disease: A prospective randomized controlled trial. *Digestion* 91 (3): 239–247.

Komulainen P, Kivipelto M, Lakka TA, et al. (2010). Exercise, fitness and cognition—A randomised controlled trial in older individuals: The DR's EXTRA study. *European Geriatric Medicine* 1 (5): 266–272.

Krikorian R, Shidler MD, Nash TA, et al. (2010). Blueberry supplementation improves memory in older adults. *Journal of Agricultural and Food Chemistry* 58 (7): 3996–4000.

Kwok TC, Lam KC, Wong PS, et al. (2011). Effectiveness of coordination exercise in improving cognitive function in older adults: A prospective study. *Clinical Interventions in Aging* 6: 261–267.

Lam LC, Chau RC, Wong BM, et al. (2012). A 1-year randomized controlled trial comparing mind body exercise (Tai Chi) with stretching and toning exercise on cognitive function in older Chinese adults at risk of cognitive decline. *Journal of the American Medical Directors Association* 13 (6): 568.e15–20.

Lee J, Pase M, Pipingas A, et al. (2015). Switching to a 10-day Mediterranean-style diet improves mood and cardiovascular function in a controlled crossover study. *Nutrition* 31 (5): 647–652.

Lees C, and Hopkins J. (2013). Effect of aerobic exercise on cognition, academic achievement, and psychosocial function in children: A systematic review of randomized control trials. *Preventing Chronic Disease* 10: E174.

Li L, Men WW, Chang YK, et al. (2014). Acute aerobic exercise increases cortical activity during working memory: A functional MRI study in female college students. *PLoS One* 9 (6): e99222.

Lichtwark IT, Newnham ED, Robinson SR, et al. (2014). Cognitive impairment in coeliac disease improves on a gluten-free diet and correlates with histological and serological indices of disease severity. *Alimentary Pharmacology & Therapeutics* 40 (2): 160–170.

Liu-Ambrose T, Donaldson MG, Ahamed Y, et al. (2008). Otago home-based strength and balance retraining improves executive functioning in older fallers: A randomized controlled trial. *Journal of the American Geriatrics Society* 56 (10): 1821–1830.

Liu-Ambrose T, Nagamatsu LS, Graf P, et al. (2010). Resistance training and executive functions: A 12-month randomized controlled trial. *Archives of Internal Medicine* 170 (2): 170–178.

Liu-Ambrose T, Nagamatsu LS, Voss MW, et al. (2012). Resistance training and functional plasticity of the aging brain: A 12-month randomized controlled trial. *Neurobiology of Aging* 33 (8): 1690–1698.

Llewellyn DJ, Lang IA, Langa KM, et al. (2010). Vitamin D and risk of cognitive decline in elderly persons. *Archives of Internal Medicine* 170 (13): 1135–1141.

Lounsbury H. (2014). *Fix Your Mood With Food: The "Live Natural, Live Well" Approach to Whole Body Health*. Guilford, CT: Globe Pequot Press.

Lupien SJ, Fiocco A, Wan N, et al. (2005). Stress hormones and human memory function across the lifespan. *Psychoneuroendocrinology* 30 (3): 225–242.

Masento NA, Golightly M, Field DT, et al. (2014). Effects of hydration status on cognitive performance and mood. *British Journal of Nutrition* 111 (10): 1841–1852.

Mayer EA, Knight R, Mazmanian SK, et al. (2014). Gut microbes and the brain: Paradigm shift in neuroscience. *Journal of Neuroscience* 34 (46): 15490–15496.

McKean J, Naug H, Nikbakht E, et al. (2016). Probiotics and subclinical psychological symptoms in healthy participants: A systematic review and meta-analysis. *Journal of Alternative and Complementary Medicine*. Electronic publication ahead of print.

Miller KJ, Dye RV, Kim J, et al. (2013). Effect of a computerized brain exercise program on cognitive performance in older adults. *American Journal of Geriatric Psychiatry* 21 (7): 655–663.

Miller KJ, Siddarth P, Gaines JM, et al. (2012). The memory fitness program: Cognitive effects of a healthy aging intervention. *American Journal of Geriatric Psychiatry* 20 (6): 514–523.

Moss M, Hewitt S, Moss L, et al. (2008). Modulation of cognitive performance and mood by aromas of peppermint and ylang-ylang. *International Journal of Neuroscience* 118 (1): 59–77.

Nagai M, Hoshide S, and Kario K. (2010). Hypertension and dementia. *American Journal of Hypertension* 23 (2): 116–124.

Nanda B, Balde J, and Manjunatha S. (2013). The acute effects of a single bout of moderate-intensity aerobic exercise on cognitive functions in healthy adult males. *Journal of Clinical and Diagnostic Research* 7 (9): 1883–1885.

Narme P, Clément S, Ehrlé N, et al. (2013). Efficacy of musical interventions in dementia: Evidence from a randomized controlled trial. *Journal of Alzheimer's Disease* 38 (2): 359–369.

Nemani K, Hosseini Ghomi R, McCormick B, et al. (2015). Schizophrenia and the gut-brain axis. *Prognosis in Neuropsychopharmacol & Biological Psychiatry* 56: 155–160.

Ng TP, Chiam PC, Lee T, et al. (2006). Curry consumption and cognitive function in the elderly. *American Journal of Epidemiology* 164 (9): 898–906

Ozkaya GY, Aydin H, Toraman FN, et al. (2005). Effect of strength and endurance training on cognition in older people. *Journal of Sports Science and Medicine* 4 (3): 300–313.

Perrig-Chiello P, Perrig WJ, Ehrsam R, et al. (1998). The effects of resistance training on well-being and memory in elderly volunteers. *Age and Ageing* 27 (4): 469–475.

Pettersen JA, Fontes S, and Duke CL. (2014). The effects of vitamin D insufficiency and seasonal decrease on cognition. *Canadian Journal of Neurological Sciences* 41 (4): 459–465.

Phillips C, Akif Baktir M, Das D, et al. (2015). The link between physical activity and cognitive dysfunction in Alzheimer disease. *Physical Therapy* 95 (7): 1046–1060.

Pierce C, Pecen J, and McLeod KJ. (2009). Influence of seated rocking on blood pressure in the elderly: A pilot clinical study. *Biological Research for Nursing* 11 (2): 144–151.

Pietrzak RH, Scott JC, Neumeister A, et al. (2014). Anxiety symptoms, cerebral amyloid burden and memory decline in healthy older adults without dementia: 3-year prospective cohort study. *British Journal of Psychiatry* 204: 400–401.

Pinniger R, Brown RF, Thorsteinsson, et al. (2012). Argentine tango dance compared to mindfulness meditation and a waiting-list control: A randomised trial for treating depression. *Complementary Therapies in Medicine* 20 (6): 377–384.

Pontifex MB, Hillman CH, Fernhall B, et al. (2009). The effect of acute aerobic and resistance exercise on working memory. *Medicine and Science in Sports and Exercise* 41 (4): 927–934.

Poon L, Chodzko-Zajko W, and Tomporowski P. (2006). *Active Living, Cognitive Functioning, and Aging* (Volume 1). Champaign IL: Human Kinetics.

Rampersaud GC, Pereira MA, Girard BL, et al. (2005). Breakfast habits, nutritional status, body weight, and academic performance in children and adolescents. *Journal of the American Dietetic Association* 105 (5): 743–760.

Roberts RO, Knopman DS, Przybelski SA, et al. (2014). Association of type 2 diabetes with brain atrophy and cognitive impairment. *Neurology* 82 (13): 1132–1141.

Sabia S, Elbaz A, Britton A, et al. (2014). Alcohol consumption and cognitive decline in early old age. *Neurology* 82 (4): 332–339.

Seamans KM, Hill TR, Scully L, et al. (2010). Vitamin D status and measures of cognitive function in healthy older European adults. *European Journal of Clinical Nutrition* 64 (10): 1172–1178.

Scott KP, Antoine JM, Midtvedt T, et al. (2015). Manipulating the gut microbiota to maintain health and treat disease. *Microbial Ecology in Health and Disease* 26: 25877.

Severance EG, Prandovszky E, Castiglione J, et al. (2015). Gastroenterology issues in schizophrenia: Why the gut matters. *Current Psychiatry Reports* 17 (5): 574.

Sharon G, Garg N, Debelius J, et al. (2014). Specialized metabolites from the microbiome in health and disease. *Cell Metabolism* 20 (5): 719–730.

Slavin J. (2013). Fiber and prebiotics: Mechanisms and health benefits. *Nutrients* 5 (4): 1417–1435.

Small G, and Vorgan G. (2004). *The Memory Prescription: Dr. Gary Small's 14-Day Plan to Keep Your Brain and Body Young.* New York, NY: Hyperion.

Small GW, Silverman DH, Siddarth P, et al. (2006). Effects of a 14-day healthy longevity lifestyle program on cognition and brain function. *American Journal of Geriatric Psychiatry* 14 (6): 538–545.

Smyth A, Dehghan, M, O'Donnell M, et al. (2015). Healthy eating and reduced risk of cognitive decline: A cohort from 40 countries. *Neurology* 84 (22): 2258–2265.

Somer E. (1999). *Food & Mood: The Complete Guide to Eating Well and Feeling Your Best*, 2nd ed. New York, NY: Henry Holt and Company.

Sompo Japan Research Institute. (2010). A non-profit organization, community health promotion support meeting "one to three" and its health promotion activities for the elderly using the FUMANET exercise. Disease Management Reporter in Japan 18: 1–8. www.sj-ri.co.jp/eng/disease/pdf/eng_dmr-18.pdf

Spirduso W, Poon L, and Chodzko-Zajko W. (2008). *Exercise and Its Mediating Effects on Cognition* (Volume 2). Champaign IL: Human Kinetics.

Swanson GR, Sedghi S, Farhadi A, et al, (2010). Pattern of alcohol consumption and its effect on gastrointestinal symptoms in inflammatory bowel disease. *Alcohol* 44 (3): 223–228.

Taibi A, and Comelli EM. (2014). Practical approaches to probiotics use. *Applied Physiology, Nutrition, and Metabolism* 39 (8): 980–986.

ten Brinke LF, Bolandzadeh N, Nagamatsu LS, et al. (2015). Aerobic exercise increases hippocampal volume in older women with probable mild cognitive impairment: A 6-month randomised controlled trial. *British Journal of Sports Medicine* 49 (4): 248–254.

Tomporowski PD, Davis CL, Miller PH, et al. (2008). Exercise and children's intelligence, cognition, and academic achievement. *Educational Psychology Review* 20 (2): 111–131.

Tsutsumi T, Don BM, Zaichkowsky LD, et al. (1997). Physical fitness and psychological benefits of strength training in community dwelling older adults. *Applied Human Science* 16 (6): 257–266.

Valls-Pedret C., Sala-Vila A., Serra-Mir M, et al. (2015). Mediterranean diet and age-related cognitive decline: A randomized clinical trial. *JAMA Internal Medicine* 175 (7): 1094–1103.

Venes D. (Ed.). (2013). *Taber's Cyclopedic Medical Dictionary*, 22nd ed. Philadelphia, PA: FA Davis.

Voss MW, Prakash RS, Erickson KI, et al. (2010). Plasticity of brain networks in a randomized intervention trial of exercise training in older adults. *Frontiers in Aging Neuroscience* 2: 32.

Weinstein G, Maillard P, Himali JJ, et al. (2015). Glucose indices are associated with cognitive and structural brain measures in young adults. *Neurology* 84 (23): 2329–2337.

Wells RE, Yeh GY, Kerr CE, et al. (2013). Meditation's impact on default mode network and hippocampus in mild cognitive impairment: A pilot study. *Neuroscience Letter* 556: 15–19.

White BA, Horwath CC, and Conner TS. (2013). Many apples a day keep the blues away—Daily experiences of negative and positive affect and food consumption in young adults. *British Journal of Health Psychology* 18 (4): 782–798.

Wilker EH, Preis SR, Beiser AS, et al. (2015). Long-term exposure to fine particulate matter, residential proximity to major roads and measures of brain structure. *Stroke* 46 (5): 1161–1166.

Winter B, Breitenstein C, Mooren FC, et al. (2007). High impact running improves learning. *Neurobiology of Learning and Memory* 87 (4): 597–609.

Wu CT, Pontifex MB, Raine LB, et al. (2011). Aerobic fitness and response variability in preadolescent children performing a cognitive control task. *Neuropsychology* 25 (3): 333–341.

Ybarra O, Burnstein E, Winkielman P, et al. (2008). Mental exercising through simple socializing: Social interaction promotes general cognitive functioning. *Personality & Social Psychology Bulletin* 34 (2): 248–259.

Yoo SS, Hu PT, Gujar N, et al. (2007). A deficit in the ability to form new human memories without sleep. *Nature Neuroscience* 10 (3): 385–392.

Young H, and Benton D. (2014). The nature of the control of blood glucose in those with poorer glucose tolerance influences mood and cognition. *Metabolic Brain Disease* 29 (3): 721–728.

Zeidan F, Martucci KT, Kraft RA, et al. (2014). Neural correlates of mindfulness meditation-related anxiety relief. *Social Cognitive and Affective Neuroscience* 9 (6): 751–759.

Zhao E, Tranovich MJ, and Wright VJ. (2014). The role of mobility as a protective factor of cognitive functioning in aging adults: A review. *Sports Health* 6 (1): 63–69.

Zhou L, and Foster JA. (2015). Psychobiotics and the gut-brain axis: In the pursuit of happiness. *Neuropsychiatric Disease and Treatment* 11: 715–723.

Zhu N, Jacobs DR, Schreiner PJ, et al. (2014). Cardiorespiratory fitness and cognitive function in middle age: The CARDIA study. *Neurology* 82 (15): 1339–1346.

PART 7

Yoga

Yoga is a system of traditional Hindu beliefs and activities thought to have originated around 3000 BC. Some teach that yoga is the skill of "effortless effort." In the Western world, yoga is primarily associated with physical postures and coordinated diaphragmatic breathing and less with its meditative aspects (Venes 2013). Yoga improves flexibility, strength, and balance, and promotes relaxation. There are many types of traditional yoga, such as Ashtanga, Bikram, Hatha, Iyengar, Kundalini, and restorative, as well as some newer variations, like Acroyoga, Anusara, and power yoga.

Why Do Yoga?

- Relieve stress and tension
- Improve overall health
- Improve flexibility
- Improve breathing
- Improve strength
- Improve balance
- Improve posture
- Improve circulation
- Help manage pain
- Help prevent falls
- Help manage weight
- Help find inner peace

Research says...

- A study in *JAMA* by Cherkin et al. (2016) found that "Among adults with chronic low back pain, treatment with mindfulness-based stress reduction (MSRB) [training in mindfulness meditation and yoga] or cognitive behavioral therapy (CBT), compared with usual care, resulted in greater improvement in back pain and functional limitations at 26 weeks, with no significant differences in outcomes between MBSR and CBT. These findings suggest that mindfulness-based stress reduction may be an effective treatment option for patients with chronic low back pain."
- A review study by Andronis et al. (2016) concluded that "The identified evidence suggests that combined physical and psychological treatments, medical yoga, information and education programmes, spinal manipulation and acupuncture are likely to be cost-effective options for low back pain."
- A review study by Chang et al. (2016) concluded that "With few exceptions, previous studies and the recent randomized control trials indicate that yoga can reduce pain and disability, can be practiced safely, and is well received by participants. Some studies also indicate that yoga may improve psychological symptoms, but these effects are currently not as well established."
- A study by Telles et al. (2016) found that "Within 12 weeks, yoga practice reduced pain and state anxiety but did not alter MRI-proven changes in the intervertebral discs and in the vertebrae."
- "High-intensity yoga may have positive effects on blood lipids and an anti-inflammatory effect" (Papp et al. 2016).
- "Yoga can effectively reduce breast cancer survivors' cognitive complaints and prompt further research on mind-body and physical activity interventions for improving cancer-related cognitive problems" (Derry et al. 2015).
- A study by Aboagye et al. (2015) found that "Six weeks of uninterrupted medical yoga therapy is a cost-effective early intervention for non-specific low back pain, when treatment recommendations are adhered to."
- A study by Monro et al. (2015) found that "Yoga therapy can be safe and beneficial for patients with nsLBP [nonspecific low back pain] or sciatica, accompanied by disc extrusions and bulges."

- A study by Nambi et al. (2014) found that "These results suggest that Iyengar yoga provides better improvement in pain reduction and improvement in HRQOL [health related quality of life] in nonspecific chronic back pain than general exercise."
- A study by Fishman et al. (2014) found that "Asymmetrically strengthening the convex side of the primary curve with daily practice of the side plank pose held for as long as possible for an average of 6.8 months significantly reduced the angle of primary scoliotic curves."
- A study by Stein et al. (2014) found that "Poor physical health at baseline is associated with greater improvement from yoga in back-related function and pain. Race, income, and body mass index do not affect the potential for a person with low back pain to experience benefit from yoga."
- Yoga can lead to possible improvements in psychological health in older adults (Bonura et al. 2014).
- Yoga is a helpful adjunct with pharmacological treatment to improve quality of life in individuals with bronchial asthma (Sodhi et al. 2014).
- Yoga may lead to improvements in cognitive function (Gothe et al. 2014; Hariprasad et al. 2013).
- Yoga has a beneficial effect on inflammatory activity and improvement in fatigue among breast-cancer survivors (Bower et al. 2012, 2014).
- Yoga is a useful addition to a school routine to boost social self-esteem (Telles et al. 2013).
- Yoga as a part of health education classes can inform about activities (Conboy et al. 2013), and provide workshops on anti-bullying, stress management, anxiety prevention techniques, and managing negative emotions.
- Hatha yoga postures performed by older adults in a study by Salem et al (2013) found that "Our findings demonstrated that Hatha yoga postures engendered a range of appreciable joint angles, joint movements of force (JMOFs), and muscle activities about the ankle, knee, and hip, and that demands associated with some postures and posture modifications were not always intuitive."
- The Yoga Empowers Seniors Study (YESS) uses "biomechanics and physical performance tests to acquire information about the physical demands placed on the muscles and joints by the asanas and the functional performance adaptations resulting from the yoga practice" (Greendale et al. 2012).
- Yoga can improve upper-extremity function in individuals with hyperkyphosis, a spine deformity that causes a forward-curved posture of the upper back

(Wang et al. 2012) and decreased adult onset kyphosis in seniors (Greendale et al. 2009).

- Yoga helps with stress control (Kiecolt-Glaser et al. 2010).
- Yoga is a helpful way to manage fear of falls and improve balance (Schmidd et al. 2010).
- Yoga can be an effective strategy to help breast-cancer survivors improve quality of life (Speed-Andrews et al. 2010).
- Yoga training in the preseason or as a supplemental activity may lessen the symptoms associated with muscle soreness (Boyle et al. 2004).
- In a preliminary study, "a yoga-based regimen was more effective than wrist splinting or no treatment in relieving some symptoms and signs of carpal tunnel syndrome" (Garfinkel et al. 1998).

Additional Resources

- International Association of Yoga Therapists, www.iayt.org
- MediYoga, http://en.mediyoga.com
- Yoga Alliance, www.yogaalliance.org
- *Yoga* journal, www.yogajournal.com
- Yogathology with Romy Phillips, http://yogathology.com

References

Aboagye E, Karlsson ML, Hagberg J, et al. (2015). Cost-effectiveness of early interventions for non-specific low back pain: A randomized controlled study investigating medical yoga, exercise therapy and self-care advice. *Journal of Rehabilitation Medicine* 47 (2): 167-173.

Andronis L, Kinghorn P, Qiao S, et al. (2016). Cost-effectiveness of non-invasive and non-pharmacological interventions for low back pain: A systematic literature review. *Applied Health Economics and Health Policy*. Electronic publication ahead of print.

Bonura KB, and Tenenbaum G. (2014). Effects of yoga on psychological health in older adults. Journal of Physical Activity & Health 11 (7): 1334–1341.

Bower JE, Garet D, Sternlieb B, et al. (2012). Yoga for persistent fatigue in breast cancer survivors: A randomized controlled trial. *Cancer* 118 (15): 3766–3775.

Bower JE, Greendale G, Crosswell AD, et al. (2014). Yoga reduces inflammatory signaling in fatigued breast cancer survivors: A randomized controlled trial. *Psychoneuroendocrinology* 43:20–29.

Chang DG, Holt JA, Sklar M, et al. (2016). Yoga as a treatment for chronic low back pain: A systematic review of the literature. *Journal of Orthopedics and Rheumatology* 3(1): 1-8.

Cherkin DC, Sherman KJ, Balderson BH, et al. (2016). Effect of mindfulness-based stress reduction vs cognitive behavioral therapy or usual care on back pain and functional limitations in adults with chronic low back pain: A randomized clinical trial. *JAMA* 315 (12): 1240-1249.

Davis CM. (2009). *Complementary Therapies in Rehabilitation: Evidence for Efficacy in Therapy, Prevention and Wellness,* 3rd ed. Thorofare, NJ: SLACK.

Derry HM, Jaremka LM, Bennett JM, et al. (2015). Yoga and self-reported cognitive problems in breast cancer survivors: A randomized controlled trial. *Psychooncology* 24 (8): 958-966.

Evans-Wentz WY. (1967). *Tibetan Yoga and Secret Doctrines.* New York, NY: Oxford University Press.

Fishman LM, Groessl EJ, Sherman KJ. (2014). Serial case reporting yoga for idiopathic and degenerative scoliosis. *Global Advances in Health and Medicine* 3 (5): 16-21.

Garfinkel MS, Singhal A, Katz WA, et al. (1998). Yoga-based intervention for carpal tunnel syndrome: A randomized trial. *JAMA* 280 (18): 1601-1603.

Greendale GA, Huang MH, Karlamangla AS, et al. (2009). Yoga decreases kyphosis in senior women and men with adult-onset hyperkyphosis: Results of a randomized controlled trial. *Journal of the American Geriatrics Society* 57 (9): 1569–1579.

Kiecolt-Glaser JK, Christian L, Preston H, et al. (2010). Stress, inflammation, and yoga practice. *Psychosomatic Medicine* 72 (2): 113–121.

Monro R, Bhardwaj AK, Gupta RK, et al. (2015). Disc extrusions and bulges in nonspecific low back pain and sciatica: Exploratory randomised controlled trial comparing yoga therapy and normal medical treatment. *Journal of Back and Musculoskeletal Rehabilitation* 28 (2): 383-392.

Nambi GS, Inbasekaran D, Khuman R, et al. (2014). Changes in pain intensity and health related quality of life with iyengar yoga in nonspecific chronic low back pain: A randomized controlled study. *International Journal of Yoga* 7 (1): 48-53.

Papp ME, Lindfors P, Nygren-Bonnier M, et al. (2016). Effects of high-intensity hatha yoga on cardiovascular fitness, adipocytokines, and apolipoproteins in healthy students: A randomized controlled study. *Journal of Alternative and Complementary Medicine* 22 (1): 81-87.

Salem G.J, Yu SS, Wang MY, et al. (2013). Physical demand profiles of hatha yoga postures performed by older adults. *Evidence-based Complementary and Alternative Medicine* 165763.

Schmidd AA, Van Puymbroeck M, and Koceja DM. (2010). Effect of a 12-week yoga intervention on fear of falling and balance in older adults: A pilot study. *Archives of Physical Medicine and Rehabilitation* 91 (4): 576–583.

Sodhi C, Singh S, and Bery A. (2014). Assessment of the quality of life in patients with bronchial asthma, before and after yoga: A randomised trial. Iranian Journal of Allergy, Asthma, and Immunology 13 (1): 55–60.

Speed-Andrews AE, Stevinson C, Belanger LJ, et al. (2010). Pilot evaluation of an Iyengar yoga program for breast cancer survivors. Cancer Nursing 33 (5): 369–381.

Stein KM, Weinberg J, Sherman KJ, et al. (2014). Participant characteristics associated with symptomatic improvement from yoga for chronic low back pain. *Journal of Yoga and Physical Therapy* 4 (1): 151.

Telles S, Bhardwaj AK, Gupta RK, et al. (2016). A randomized controlled trial to assess pain and magnetic resonance imaging-based (MRI-based) structural spine changes in low back pain patients after yoga practice. *Medical Science Monitor* 22: 3228-3247.

Telles S, Singh N, Bhardwaj AK et al. (2013). Effect of yoga or physical exercise on physical, cognitive and emotional measures in children: A randomized controlled trial. Child and Adolescent Psychiatry and Mental Health 7 (1): 37.

Venes D. (Ed.) (2013). Taber's Cyclopedic Medical Dictionary, 22nd ed. Philadelphia, PA: FA Davis.

Wang MY, Greendale GA, Kazadi L, et al. (2012). Yoga improves upper-extremity function and scapular posturing in persons with hyperkyphosis. *Journal of Yoga and Physical Therapy* 2 (3): 117.

Wang MY, Yu SS, Hashish R, et al. (2013). The biomechanical demands of standing yoga poses in seniors: The Yoga Empowers Seniors Study (YESS). BMC Complementary and Alternative Medicine 13:

PART 8

Tai Chi

Tai chi is a traditional Chinese martial art in which a series of slow, controlled movements helps improve balance, relaxation, mental concentration, flexibility, and strength (Venes 2013). Tai chi is sometimes considered mind in action or meditation in motion (Chow 1982).

The exact origin of tai chi is unknown. Chinese legend has it that it began about 800 years ago, when a Taoist priest named Zhang Sanfeng witnessed a fight between a bird and a snake. He became fascinated by the fluid motions both animals used in going from offense to defense. Over a period of several years, he experimented with various forms until he developed what is now practiced as tai chi.

Today there are several styles of tai chi, such as the Yang, Chen, Wu, Hao, and Sun styles, with some forms having more than 100 postures and movements. Traditional styles are associated with family surnames: Chen, Yang (most popular form), Wu, and Sun (Kit 2002).

Why Do Tai Chi?

- Relieve stress and tension
- Improve overall health
- Improve flexibility
- Improve breathing
- Improve strength
- Improve posture
- Improve balance
- Improve circulation

- Help manage pain
- Help prevent falls
- Help manage weight
- Help find inner peace

Research says...

- Tai chi may be a good way to slow down the age-related decline in muscle strength in a community-dwelling population (Zhou et al. 2016).
- Tai chi can be helpful for improving fitness and arthritis in older adults (Dogra et al. 2015).
- Tai chi and functional balance training benefit older individuals with poly-neuropathy (Quigley et al. 2014).
- Tai chi has had modest positive effects on functional status of individuals with Parkinson's disease (Choi et al. 2013; Li et al. 2012).
- Speed and accuracy in math computations has been attributed to the possible relaxed state from a tai chi or yoga class (Field et al. 2010).
- Tai chi can improve the quality of life for individuals with chronic obstructive pulmonary disease (COPD) (Yeh et al. 2010).
- Tai chi can be useful in the treatment of fibromyalgia (Wang et al. 2010).
- Tai chi can lead to balance improvements in people with chronic strokes (Au-Yeung et al. 2009).
- Tai chi improves balance and helps people maintain good postural stability (Li et al. 2008; Mak et al. 2003, Tsang et al. 2004).
- Tai chi can be beneficial for reducing falls (Li et al. 2005; Voukelatos 2007).
- Tai chi can improve sleep quality in older adults (Li et al. 2004).
- Tai chi has been shown to slow the loss of weight-bearing bone in postmeno-pausal women (Chan et al. 2004; Qin et al. 2002).
- Tai chi can improve a person's arthritic symptoms (Song et al. 2003).
- Tai chi can have a positive effect on immunity that protects against shingles (Irwin et al. 2003).

Additional Resources

- American Tai Chi and Qigong Association, www.americantaichi.org
- International Sun Tai Chi Association, www.suntaichi.com

References

Au-Yeung SS, Hui-Chan CW, and Tang JC. (2009). Short-form Tai Chi improves standing balance of people with chronic stroke. *Neurorehabilitation and Neural Repair* 23 (5): 515–522.

Chan K, Qin L, Lau M, et al. (2004). A randomized prospective study of the effects of Tai Chi Chun exercise on bone mineral density in postmenopausal women. *Archives of Physical Medicine and Rehabilitation* 85 (5): 717–722.

Choi HJ, Garber CE, Jun TW, et al. (2013). Therapeutic effects of Tai Chi in patients with Parkinson's disease. *ISRN Neurology* 548240.

Chow M. (1982). *Classical Yang Style Tai Chi Chuan.* Los Angeles, CA: Wen Lin Associates.

Davis CM. (2009). *Complementary Therapies in Rehabilitation: Evidence for Efficacy in Therapy, Prevention and Wellness,* 3rd ed. Thorofare, NJ: SLACK.

Dogra S, Shah S, Patel M, et al. (2015). Effectiveness of a tai chi intervention for improving functional fitness and general health among ethnically diverse older adults with self-reported arthritis living in low-income neighborhoods: A cohort study. *Journal of Geriatric Physical Therapy* 38 (2): 71–77.

Field T, Diego M, and Hernandez-Reif M. (2010). Tai chi/yoga effects on anxiety, heartrate, EEG and math computations. *Complementary Therapies in Clinical Practice* 16 (4): 235–238.

Irwin MR, Pike JL, Cole JC, et al. (2003). Effects of a behavioral intervention, Tai Chi Chih, on varicella-zoster virus specific immunity and health functioning in older adults. *Psychosomatic Medicine* 65 (5): 824–830.

Kit WA. (2002). *The Complete Book of Tai Chi Chuan.* Boston, MA: Tuttle Publishing.

Li F, Fisher KJ, Harmer P, et al. (2004). Tai chi and self-rated quality of sleep and daytime sleepiness in older adults: a randomized controlled trial. *Journal of the American Geriatrics Society* 52 (6): 892–900.

Li F, Harmer P, Fisher KJ, et al. (2005). Tai chi and fall reductions in older adults: a randomized controlled trial. *Journals of Gerontology; Series A; Biological Sciences and Medical Sciences* 60 (2): 187–194.

Li F, Harmer P, Fitzgerald K, et al. (2012). Tai chi and postural stability in patients with Parkinson's disease. *New England Journal of Medicine* 366 (6): 511–519.

Li JX, Xu DQ, and Hong Y. (2008). Effects of 16-week Tai Chi intervention on postural stability and proprioception of knee and ankle in older people. *Age and Ageing* 37 (5): 575–578.

Mak MK, and Ng PL. (2003). Mediolateral sway in single-leg stance is the best discriminator of balance performance for tai-chi practitioners. *Archives of Physical Medicine and Rehabilitation* 84 (5): 683–686.

Qin L, Au S, Choy W, et al. (2002). Regular Tai Chi Chuan exercise may retard bone loss in postmenopausal women: a case-control study. *Archives of Physical Medicine and Rehabilitation* 83 (10): 1355–1359.

Quigley PA, Bulat T, Schulz B, et al. (2014). Exercise interventions, gait, and balance in older subjects with distal symmetric polyneuropathy: a three-group randomized clinical trial. American Journal of Physical Medicine and Rehabilitation 93 (1): 1–16.

Song R, Lee EO, Lam P, et al. (2003). Effects of Tai Chi exercise on pain, balance, muscle strength, and perceived difficulties in physical functioning in older women with osteoarthritis: a randomized clinical trial. Journal of Rheumatology 30 (9): 2039–2044.

Tsang WW, and Hui-Chan CW. (2004). Effects of exercise on joint sense and balance in elderly men: Tai Chi versus golf. *Medicine & Science in Sports & Exercise* 36 (4): 658–667.

Venes D. (Ed.) (2013). Taber's Cyclopedic Medical Dictionary, 22nd ed. Philadelphia, PA: FA Davis.

Voukelatos A, Cumming RG, Lord SR, et al. (2007). A randomized, controlled trial of Tai Chi for the prevention of falls: the Central Sydney Tai Chi trial. Journal of the American Geriatrics Society 55 (8): 1185–1191.

Wang C, Schmid CH, Rones R, et al. (2010). A randomized trial of Tai Chi for fibromyalgia. New England Journal of Medicine 363 (8): 743–754.

Yeh GY, Roberts DH, Wayne PM, et al. (2010). Tai chi exercise for patients with chronic obstructive pulmonary disease: a pilot study. Respiratory Care 55 (11): 1475–1482.

Zhou M, Peng N, Dai Q, et al. (2016). Effect of tai chi on muscle strength of the lower extremities in the elderly. *Chinese Journal of Integrative Medicine* 22 (11): 861-866.

PART 9

Qi Gong

Qigong is a traditional Chinese movement therapy (Kerr 2002) and ancient martial art approach to healing that harnesses internal energy through movement (postures involving strength, flexibility, and balance), breathing exercises, relaxation, and meditation. *Qi* (breath, air, spirit) in Chinese stands for "energy of life" and *gong* means "work" or "practice." Thus, *qigong* means "working with the energy of life" (Johnson 2000; Venes 2013).

The word "qigong" dates back to two published works, in 1915 and 1929, and the therapeutic use of the term dates to 1936. Common use of the term is relatively recent as the practice has been known by many names throughout Chinese history, such as chi kung. There are many forms of qigong, such as Medical Qigong, Fragrant Qigong, Guo Lin Qigong (walking qigong), Five Animals Play Qigong, Eight Strands of Brocade Qigong, Tai Chi Qigong, and Six Healing Sounds. Also, qigong has several schools with their unique theories, such as Chinese Medical Qigong, Daoist Qigong, Buddhist Qigong, Confucian Qigong, and Martial Arts Qigong. The earliest qigong-like exercises in China are ritual animal dances and movements. Many qigong postures have names such as Bathing Duck, Leaping Monkey, Turning Tiger, Coiling Snake, Old Bear in the Woods, and Flying Crane (Cohen 1997).

Why Do Qi Gong?

- Relieve stress and tension
- Improve overall health

- Improve flexibility
- Improve breathing
- Improve strength
- Improve balance
- Improve posture
- Improve circulation
- Help manage pain
- Help manage weight
- Help find inner peace

Research says...

- Tai Chi Qigong is useful for improving the quality of sleep in older adults with cognitive impairment (Chan et al 2016).
- Qigong has been shown to be influential to postural stability and Parkinson's disease-related falls (Loftus 2014).
- A study by Fong et al. (2015) found that "TC [tai chi] Qigong could be an effective nonpharmacological intervention for managing progressive trismus [tonic contraction of the muscles of mastication], chronic neck and shoulder hypomobility, and reducing sleep problems among nasopharyngeal cancer survivors."
- Qigong can improve balance in healthy young women (González López-Arza et al. 2013).
- Qigong can improve psychosocial health in individuals with chronic obstructive pulmonary disease (COPD) (Chan et al. 2013).
- Qigong has shown to cause short-term improvement of quality of life, pain, and sleep quality in individuals diagnosed with fibromyalgia (Lauche et al. 2013).
- Qigong can reduce chronic neck pain (Rendant et al. 2011).
- Qigong can decrease blood pressure in individuals with essential hypertension, which develops with no apparent cause (Guo et al. 2008).
- Qigong can help reduce pain and anxiety in individuals with complex regional pain syndrome (Wu et al. 1999).
- Qigong helps elderly individuals with chronic physical and mental illness (Tsang et al. 2003).

Additional Resources

- American Tai Chi and Qigong Association, www.americantaichi.org
- National Qigong Association, http://nqa.org
- Qigong Institute, www.qigonginstitute.org

References

Chan AW, Yu DS, Choi KC, et al. (2016). Tai chi qigong as a means to improve night-time sleep quality among older adults with cognitive impairment: A pilot randomized controlled trial. *Clinical Interventions in Aging* 11: 1277-1286.

Chan AW, Lee A, Lee DT, et al. (2013). Evaluation of the sustaining effects of Tai Chi qigong in the sixth month in promoting psychosocial health in COPD patients: a single-blind, randomized controlled trial. *Scientific World Journal* 425082.

Cohen KS. (1997). *The Way of Qigong: The Art and Science of Chinese Energy Healing.* New York, NY: Ballantine Books.

Davis CM. (2009). *Complementary Therapies in Rehabilitation: Evidence for Efficacy in Therapy, Prevention and Wellness,* 3rd ed. Thorofare, NJ: SLACK.

Fong SS, Ng SS, Lee HW, et al. (2015). The effects of a 6-month Tai Chi Qigong training program on temporomandibular, cervical, and shoulder joint mobility and sleep problems in nasopharyngeal cancer survivors. *Integrative Cancer Therapies* 14 (1): 16–25.

González López-Arza MV, Varela-Donoso E, Montanero-Fernandez J, et al. (2013). Qigong improves balance in young women: a pilot study. *Journal of Integrative Medicine* 11 (4): 241–245.

Guo X, Zhou B, Nishimura T, et al. (2008). Clinical effect of qigong practice on essential hypertension: a meta-analysis of randomized controlled trials. *Journal of Alternative and Complementary Medicine* 14 (1): 27–37.

Johnson JA. (2000). *Chinese Medical Qigong Therapy: A Comprehensive Clinical Text.* International Institute of Medical Qigong. Pacific Grove, CA.

Kerr C. (2002). Translating "mind-in-body": two models of patient experience underlying a randomized controlled trial of qigong. *Culture, Medicine and Psychiatry* 26 (4): 419–447.

Lauche R, Cramer H, Hauser W. et al. (2013). A systematic review and meta-analysis of qigong for the fibromyalgia syndrome. *Evidence-Based Complementary and Alternative Medicine* 635182.

Liu MH, and Perry P. (1997). *The Healing Art of Qi Gong.* New York, NY: Warner Books.

Loftus S. (2014). Qi Gong to improve postural stability for Parkinson fall prevention: A neuroplasticity approach. *Topics in Geriatric Rehabilitation* 30 (1): 58–69.

Rendant D, Pach D, Lüdtke R, et al. (2011). Qigong versus exercise versus no therapy for patients with chronic neck pain: a randomized controlled trial. *Spine (Philadelphia, Pa. 1976)* 36 (6): 419–427.

Tsang HW, Mok CK, Au Yeung YT, et al. (2003). The effect of qigong on general and psychosocial health of elderly with chronic physical illnesses: a randomized clinical trial. *International Journal of Geriatric Psychiatry* 18 (5): 441–449.

Venes D. (Ed.) (2013). *Taber's Cyclopedic Medical Dictionary,* 22nd ed. Philadelphia, PA: FA Davis.

Wu WH, Bandilla E, Ciccone DS, et al. (1999). Effects of qigong on late-stage complex regional pain syndrome. *Alternative Therapies in Health and Medicine* 5 (1): 45–54.

PART 10
Pilates

German-born Joseph H. Pilates is the creator of the Pilates system, a form of bodywork that uses controlled movements and poses to improve strength, flexibility, balance, and mental concentration. Throughout his career, Pilates developed many original exercise machines (such as the Reformer, Cadillac, Wunda Chair, and Ladder Barrel), created a mat exercise series, wrote two books (Pilates 1934; Pilates et al. 1945), and formulated unique exercise theories.

Why Do Pilates?

- Relieve stress and tension
- Improve overall health
- Improve flexibility
- Improve breathing
- Improve overall strength
- Improve core strength
- Improve balance
- Improve posture
- Improve circulation
- Help manage weight

Research says...

- Pilates may benefit postmenopausal women with chronic low back pain (Cruz-Diaz et al. 2016).

- Pilates is effective in improving pain, flexibility, and balance in individuals with chronic non-specific low back pain (Valenza et al. 2016).
- Equipment-based Pilates may be superior to mat Pilates for disability and kinesiophobia (fear of movement) in individuals suffering from chronic lower-back pain (da Luz et al. 2014).
- Pilates may lead to decreased fall risk (Stivala et al. 2014).
- Pilates can reduce the degree of nonstructural scoliosis and increase flexibility and decrease pain (Alves de Araújo et al. 2012).
- Pilates can improve abdominal wall muscles (Dorado et al. 2012).
- Pilates can enhance functional capacity in individuals with heart failure, when combined with standard medical therapy (Guimarães et al. 2012).
- Pilates can be beneficial for disability, pain, function, and health-related quality of life (Wajswelner et al. 2012).
- Pilates improves mindfulness (changes in mood and perceived stress) (Caldwell et al. 2010).
- Pilates improves abdominal strength and upper-spine posture (Emery et al. 2010).
- Pilates is effective and safe for female breast-cancer patients (Eyigor et al. 2010).
- Pilates improves muscular endurance and flexibility (Kloubec 2010).
- Pilates is an effective and safe physical activity for individuals with fibromyalgia (Altan et al. 2009).
- Pilates improves thoracic kyphosis (Kuo et al. 2009).
- Pilates improves the leaping ability of elite rhythmic gymnasts (Hutchinson et al. 1998).

Additional Resources

- Pilates Method Alliance, www.pilatesmethodalliance.org
- Polestar Pilates Education, www.polestarpilates.com

References

Altan L, Korkmaz N, Bingol U, et al. (2009). Effect of Pilates training on people with fibro-myalgia syndrome: A pilot study. *Archives of Physical Medicine and Rehabilitation* 90 (12): 1983–1988.

Alves de Araújo ME, Bezerra da Silva E, Bragade Mello D, et al. (2012). The effectiveness of the Pilates method: Reducing the degree of non-structural scoliosis, and improving flexibility and pain in female college students. *Journal of Bodywork and Movement Therapies* 16 (2): 191–198.

Caldwell K, Harrison M, Adams M, et al. (2010). Developing mindfulness in college students through movement-based courses: Effects on self-regulatory self-efficacy, mood, stress, and sleep quality. *Journal of American College Health* 58 (5): 433–442.

Cruz-Diaz D, Martinez-Amat A, Osuna-Perez MC, et al. (2016). Short- and long-term effects of a six-week clinical pilates program in addition to physical therapy on postmenopausal women with chronic low back pain: A randomized controlled trial. *Disability and Rehabilitation* 38 (13): 1300-1308.

da Luz MA., Jr., Costa LO, Fuhro FF, et al. (2014). Effectiveness of mat Pilates or equipment-based Pilates exercises in patients with chronic nonspecific low back pain: A randomized controlled trial. *Physical Therapy* 94 (5): 623–631.

Davis CM. (2009). *Complementary Therapies in Rehabilitation: Evidence for Efficacy in Therapy, Prevention and Wellness,* 3rd ed. Thorofare, NJ: SLACK.

Dorado C, Calbet JAL, Lopez-Gordillo A, et al. (2012). Marked effects of Pilates on the abdominal muscles: A longitudinal magnetic resonance imaging study. *Medicine & Science in Sports & Exercise* 44 (8): 1589–1594.

Emery K, De Serres SJ, McMillan A, et al. (2010). The effects of a Pilates training program on arm-trunk posture and movement. *Clinical Biomechanics* 25 (2): 124–130.

Eyigor S, Karapolat H, Yesil H, et al. (2010). Effects of Pilates exercises on functional capacity, flexibility, fatigue, depression and quality of life in female breast cancer patients: A randomized controlled study. *European Journal of Physical and Rehabilitation Medicine* 46 (4): 481–487.

Guimarães GV, Carvalho VO, Bocchi EA, et al. (2012). Pilates in heart failure patients: A randomized controlled pilot trial. *Cardiovascular Therapeutics* 30 (6): 351–356.

Hutchinson MR, Tremain L, Christiansen J, et al. (1998). Improving leaping ability in elite rhythmic gymnasts. *Medicine and Science in Sports and Exercise* 30 (10): 1543–1547.

Kloubec JA. (2010). Pilates for improvement of muscle endurance, flexibility, balance, and posture. *Journal of Strength and Conditioning Research* 24 (3): 661–667.

Kuo YL, Tully EA, and Galea MP. (2009). Sagittal spinal posture after Pilates-based exercise in healthy older adults. *Spine* 34 (10): 1046–1051.

Pilates JH. (1934). *Your Health: A Corrective System of Exercising that Revolutionizes the Entire Field of Physical Education*. New York, NY: C. J. O'Brien, Inc.

Pilates JH, and Miller WJ. (1945). *Return to Life Through Contrology*. New York, NY: J.J. Augustin.

Stivala A, and Hartley G. (2014). The effects of a Pilates-based exercise rehabilitation program on functional outcome and fall risk reduction in an aging adult status-post traumatic hip fracture due to fall. *Journal of Geriatric Physical Therapy* 37 (3): 136–145.

Valenza MC, Rodriguez-Torres J, Cabrera-Martos I, et al. (2016). Results of a pilates exercise program in patients with chronic non-specific low back pain: A randomized controlled trial. *Clinical Rehabilitation*. Electronic publication ahead of print.

Wajswelner H, Metcalf B, and Bennell K. (2012). Clinical Pilates versus general exercise for chronic low back pain: Randomized trial. *Medicine & Science in Sports and Exercise* 44 (7): 1197–1205.

PART 11

Feldenkrais Method

Ukrainian-born physicist Moshe Feldenkrais is the creator of the Feldenkrais Method, a form of bodywork aimed at improving posture, increasing range of motion, and relieving stress (Venes 2013). Feldenkrais spent his lifetime exploring human movement and wrote eight books (Feldenkrais 1944, 1949, 1952, 1972, 1977, 1981, 1984, 1985). Gradually, Feldenkrais formulated his ideas into an educational method, divided into two parts: *Awareness Through Movement (ATM)* and *Functional Integration (FI)* (Reese 2002).

Awareness Through Movement lessons incorporate verbally-directed active movements, visualization, and attention for group or individual work. These lessons include developmental movements, like crawling and rolling, and functions, such as posture and breathing, as well as systematic exploration of body movements. *Functional Integration*, on the other hand, is a nonverbal, manual contact technique for those requiring more individualized attention.

Why Do the Feldenkrais Method?

- Relieve stress and tension
- Improve overall health
- Improve flexibility
- Improve breathing
- Improve posture
- Help manage pain
- Help prevent falls
- Help find inner peace

Research says...

- The Feldenkrais Method may offset age-related decline in cognitive function (Ullman et al. 2016).
- A study by Verrel et al. (2015) found that "a short, non-intrusive sensorimotor intervention based on the Feldenkrais method can have effects on spontaneous cortical activity in functionally related regions."
- A study by Lundqvist et al. (2014) indicates that the "Feldenkrais method is an effective intervention for chronic neck/scapular pain in patients with visual impairment."
- The Feldenkrais Method positively affects performance of the Four Square Step Test (a test of dynamic balance) and changes in gait in individuals with osteoarthritis (Webb et al. 2013).
- The Feldenkrais Method improves balance and mobility (Connors et al. 2010; Ullmann et al. 2010).
- The Feldenkrais Method can improve health-related quality of life in individuals with nonspecific musculoskeletal disorders (Malmgren-Olsson et al. 2002).

Additional Resources

- Feldenkrais Guild of North America, www.feldenkrais.com
- International Feldenkrais Federation, http://feldenkrais-method.org

References

Connors KA, Galea MP, and Said CM. (2010). Feldenkrais Method balance classes are based on principles of motor learning and postural control retraining: A qualitative research study. *Physiotherapy* 96 (4): 324–336.

Connors KA, Pile C, Nichols ME. (2011). Does the Feldenkrais Method make a difference? An investigation into the use of outcome measurement tools for evaluating changes in clients. *Journal of Bodywork & Movement Therapies*, 15(4), 446-52.

Davis CM. (2009). *Complementary Therapies in Rehabilitation: Evidence for Efficacy in Therapy, Prevention and Wellness,* 3rd ed. Thorofare, NJ: SLACK.

Feldenkrais M. (1944). *Judo: The Art of Defense and Attack*. New York, NY: Frederick Warne & Co.

Feldenkrais M. (1949). *Body and Mature Behaviour: A Study of Anxiety, Sex, Gravitation & Learning*. New York, NY: International Universities Press.

Feldenkrais M. (1952). *Higher Judo*. New York, NY: Frederick Warne & Co.

Feldenkrais M. (1972). *Awareness Through Movement: Health Exercises for Personal Growth*. New York, NY: Harper & Row.

Feldenkrais M. (1977). *The Case of Nora: Body Awareness as Healing Therapy*. New York, NY: Harper & Row.

Feldenkrais M. (1981). *The Elusive Obvious or Basic Feldenkrais*. Cupertino, CA: Meta Publications.

Feldenkrais M. (1984). *The Master Moves*. Cupertino, CA: Meta Publications.

Feldenkrais M, and Kimmey M. (Ed.). (1985). *The Potent Self: A Guide to Spontaneity*. San Francisco, CA: Harper & Row.

Hillier S, Worley A. (2015). The effectiveness of the Feldenkrais method: a systematic review of the evidence. *Evidence Based Complementary and Alternative Medicine* 1-12.

Jain S, Janssen K, Decelle S. (2004). Alexander technique and Feldenkrais method: a critical overview. *Physical Medicine and Rehabilitation Clinics of North America* 15 (4): 811-825.

Lake B. Acute back pain. (1985). Treatment by the application of Feldenkrais principles. *Australian Family Physician*. 14 (11): 1175-1178.

Lundqvist LO, Zetterlund C, and Richter HO. (2014). Effects of Feldenkrais method on chronic neck/scapular pain in people with visual impairment: A randomized controlled trial with one-year follow-up. *Archives of Physical Medicine and Rehabilitation* 95 (9): 1656–1661.

Malmgren-Olsson EB, and Branholm IB. (2002). A comparison between three physiotherapy approaches with regard to health-related factors in patients with non-specific musculoskeletal disorders. *Disability and Rehabilitation* 24 (6): 308–317.

Mattes J. (2016). Attentional Focus in Motor Learning, the Feldenkrais Method, and Mindful Movement. *Perceptual and Motor Skills* 123 (1): 258-76.

Myers LK. (2016). Application of neuroplasticity theory through the use of the Feldenkrais Method with a runner with scoliosis and hip and lumbar pain: A case report. *Journal of Bodywork & Movement Therapies*. 20 (2): 300-309.

Ohman A, Aström L, Malmgren-Olsson EB. (2011). Feldenkrais therapy as group treatment for chronic pain -A qualitative evaluation. *Journal of Bodywork & Movement Therapies* 15 (2):153-161.

Pugh JD, Williams AM. (2014). Feldenkrais Method empowers adults with chronic back pain. *Holistic Nursing Practice* 28 (3):171-83.

Reese M. (2002). *Moshe Feldenkrais and his methods: Historical background.* Class notes from Feldenkrais workshop. San Diego, CA: Feldenkrais Southern California Movement Institute. July 12.

Stephens J, Davidson J, Derosa J, et al. (2006). lengthening the hamstring muscles without stretching using "Awareness Through Movement." *Physical Therapy* 86 (12):1641-1650.

Teixeira-Machado L, Araújo FM, Cunha FA, et al. (2010). Feldenkrais Method-based exercise improves quality of life in individuals with Parkinson's disease: a controlled, randomized clinical trial. *Alternative Therapies Health Medicine* 21 (1): 8-14.

Ullmann G, Williams HG. (2016). The Feldenkrais Method can enhance cognitive function in independent living older adults: A case-series. *Journal of Bodywork and Movement Therapies* 20 (3): 512-517.

Ullmann G, Williams HG, Hussey J, et al. (2010). Effects of Feldenkrais exercises on balance, mobility, balance confidence, and gait performance in community-dwelling adults age 65 and older. *Journal of Alternative and Complementary Medicine* 16 (1): 97–105.

Venes D. (Ed.) (2013). Taber's Cyclopedic Medical Dictionary, 22nd ed. Philadelphia, PA: FA Davis.

Verrel J, Almagor E, Schumann F, et al. (2015). Changes in neural resting state activity in primary and higher-order motor areas induced by a short sensorimotor intervention based on the Feldenkrais method. *Frontiers in Human Neuroscience* 9: 232.

Webb R, Cofre Lizama LE, and Galea MP. (2013). Moving with ease: Feldenkrais Method classes for people with osteoarthritis. *Evidence-Based Complementary and Alternative Medicine* 479142.

PART 12

Alexander Technique

The Alexander Technique is a form of bodywork, created by Tasmanian-born Frederick M. Alexander, that promotes postural health (Venes 2013). During his career, Alexander wrote four books (Alexander 1918, 1923, 1932, 1941). Gradually, he developed an educational system that helps reeducate the whole body in proper movement patterns and postural habits. This educational method is known as the Alexander Technique.

Why do the Alexander Technique?

- Improve breathing
- Improve walking
- Improve balance
- Improve performance if you are a singer, musician, actor, or dancer

Research says...

- A study by Hamel et al. (2016) found that "older Alexander Technique (AT) practitioners walked with gait patterns more similar to those found in the literature for younger adults" and that AT may serve a role in reducing the negative changes in gait that occur with aging.
- Alexander Technique lessons and acupuncture both led to significant reductions in neck pain and disability (MacPherson et al. 2015).
- A study by Gleeson et al. (2015) indicates that "The intervention [Alexander Technique lessons] did not have a significant impact on the primary

outcomes but benefits for the intervention group in postural sway, trends towards fewer falls and injurious falls and improved mobility among past multiple-fallers."

- An article by Klein et al. (2014) suggests that "Alexander Technique sessions may improve performance anxiety in musicians."
- A study by Cacciatore et al. (2011) indicates that "Alexander Technique teachers, who undergo long-term training, and short-term Alexander Technique training in low-back pain subjects are associated with decreased axial stiffness."
- The Alexander Technique can significantly improve the posture of surgeons and surgical ergonomics and endurance, and decrease surgical fatigue and incidence of repetitive stress injuries (Reddy et al. 2011).
- A study by Little et al. (2008) indicates that "one-to-one lessons in the Alexander technique from registered teachers have long-term benefits [such as decreased back pain and improved quality of life] for patients with chronic back pain. Six lessons followed by exercise prescription were nearly as effective as 24 lessons."
- A study by Stallibrass et al. (2002) indicates that "lessons in the Alexander Technique are likely to lead to sustained benefit [such as less depression and improved activities of daily living] for people with Parkinson's disease."
- A study by Dennis (1999) indicates that Alexander Technique instruction may be helpful in improving balance in older women.

Additional Resources

- Alexander Technique International, www.ati-net.com
- American Society for the Alexander Technique, www.amsatonline.org
- The Complete Guide to the Alexander Technique, www.alexandertechnique.com

References

Alexander FM. (1918). *Man's Supreme Inheritance.* New York, NY: E. P. Dutton and Co., Inc.

Alexander FM. (1923). *Constructive Conscious Control of the Individual.* New York, NY: E. P. Dutton and Co., Inc.

Alexander FM. (1932). *The Use of the Self.* New York, NY: E. P. Dutton and Co., Inc.

Alexander FM. (1941). *The Universal Constant in Living.* New York, NY: E. P. Dutton and Co., Inc.

Cacciatore TW, Gurfinkel VS, Horak FB, et al. (2011). Increased dynamic regulation of postural tone through Alexander Technique training. *Human Movement Science* 30 (1): 74–89.

Davis CM. (2009). *Complementary Therapies in Rehabilitation: Evidence for Efficacy in Therapy, Prevention and Wellness,* 3rd ed. Thorofare, NJ: SLACK.

Dennis RJ. (1999). Functional reach improvement in normal older women after Alexander Technique instruction. *Journals of Gerontology. Series A, Biological Sciences and Medical Sciences* 54 (1): M8–11.

Gleeson M, Sherrington C, Lo S, et al. (2015). Can the Alexander Technique improve balance and mobility in older adults with visual impairments? A randomized controlled trial. *Clinical Rehabilitation* 29 (3): 244-260.

Hamel KA, Ross C, Schultz B, et al. (2016). Older adult alexander technique practitioners walk differently than healthy age-matched controls. *Journal of Bodywork and Movement Therapies* 20 (4): 751-760.

Klein SD, Bayard C, and Wolf U. (2014). The Alexander Technique and musicians: A systematic review of controlled trials. *BMC Complementary and Alternative Medicine,* 14: 414.

Little P, Lewith G, Webley F, et al. (2008). Randomised controlled trial of Alexander technique lessons, exercise, and massage (ATEAM) for chronic and recurrent back pain. *British Journal of Sports Medicine* 42 (12): 965–968.

MacPherson H, Tilbrook H, Richmond S, et al. (2015). Alexander technique lessons or acupuncture sessions for persons with chronic neck pain: A randomized trial. *Annals of Internal Medicine* 163 (9): 653-662.

Reddy PP, Reddy TP, Roig-Francoli J, et al. (2011). The impact of the Alexander Technique on improving posture and surgical ergonomics during minimally invasive surgery: Pilot study. *Journal of Urology* 186 (Supplement 4): 1658–1662.

Stallibrass C, Sissons P, and Chalmers C. (2002). Randomized controlled trial of the Alexander Technique for idiopathic Parkinson's disease. *Clinical Rehabilitation* 16 (7): 695–708.

Venes D. (Ed.) (2013). *Taber's Cyclopedic Medical Dictionary,* 22nd ed. Philadelphia, PA: FA Davis.

PART 13
Mindfulness Training

RELAXATION TRAINING

Relaxation slows heart rate, decreases blood pressure, and helps reduces anxiety and pain. Try the following two time-tested adapted techniques of progressive relaxation created by pioneering psychiatrist Edmund Jacobson, MD, PhD.

Do these relaxation techniques while sitting in a chair, lying on your bed, reclining in the park on some soft grass, or relaxing at the beach (Jacobson 1962, 1964, 1964, 1967, 1976). Go *very* slowly through each two-and-a-half-minute routine, and breathe naturally. For best results, loosen tight clothing and remove shoes, lie on your back with a small towel under your lower back (if needed) with a small pillow under your knees, and close your eyes.

Relaxation Activities

- Spin a pink or blue wooden dreidel (spin clockwise and counterclockwise, alternating with the left and right hands). A dreidel is a four-sided spinning top, and in Yiddish it means "to turn around," www.dreidelstore.com
- Play with a pink or blue yo-yo, http://yomega.com
- Spin Chinese Therapy Balls in your hand, www.baodingballs.com

Additional Resources

- Carolyn McManus, PT, MS, MA, www.carolynmcmanus.com (search for Guided Relaxation & Meditation).

MINDFULNESS AND MEDITATION TRAINING

Mindfulness-based stress reduction is "the use of meditation and self-awareness to enhance one's ability to cope with challenging circumstances and psychological tensions" (Venes et al. 2013). A form of mindfulness-based stress reduction was developed by Jon Kabat-Zinn, PhD at the University of Massachusetts Medical School, Center for Mindfulness. A definition proposed by Kabat-Zinn (2003) for mindfulness meditation is "the awareness that emerges through paying attention on purpose, in the present moment, and nonjudgmentally to the unfolding of experience moment by moment."

For example, research shows that mindfulness meditation can reduce anxiety (Chen et al. 2012) and benefit some individuals with multiple sclerosis in terms of quality of life (Simpson et al. 2014). Also, combining cognitive behavioral therapy and mindfulness meditation might have long-term beneficial effects on insomnia (Ong et al. 2009).

A study by Fredrickson et al. (2008) concludes that "just as the broaden-and-build theory predicts, then, when people open their hearts to positive emotions, they seed their own growth in ways that transform them for the better."

When creating your home gym, pick a spot where you get outdoor light and fresh air. Now place a few nice plants in your space, hang some inspirational pictures, and set up a good sound system to play your favorite music. These are some potential areas for setting up a gym or fitness center in your home: garage, patio, backyard, living/dining room, spare room, basement, loft, den, sunroom, or a floor-to-ceiling bay window alcove.

FENG SHUI FOR FITNESS

Include some feng shui into your home gym or outdoor fitness gazebo to create an energizing, yet calming place for yourself. Feng shui as used in this book is not about controlling your life, but rather about giving you some guidelines to create a peaceful home-fitness environment. Ultimately, do what makes you happy and what makes sense for your personal needs. Consider the following when creating your home gym:

- Area is well lit by natural light and has good air flow
- Install a small ceiling fan for air circulation
- Have an inspiring view (such as your garden, patio, or backyard), along with art and sculptures to help you relax and reflect, and plants and flowers to enrich your environment
- Buy a fish tank for relaxation and meditation

- Pick wall and furniture colors for your goals, such as red for energy or blue for relaxation
- Use fabrics made of natural fibers
- Keep clutter to a minimum

HOME GAZEBO FOR HEALING AND HEALTH

A gazebo in your backyard (or as an extension to your house) provides shade, and it's a great way to entertain friends and family. However, you can also customize your gazebo so that it helps you heal and get fit. One study indicates that outdoor training leads to greater exercise adherence than indoor training in postmenopausal women (Lacharité-Lemieux et al. 2015). So why wait? Go outside and have some fun!

Styles

- Open gazebo (no windows)—good for warm-weather locations
- Closed gazebo (windows and screens)—good for cold-weather locations

Purpose

- Fitness
- Healing
- Meditation
- Relaxation
- Body-based exercise, such as tai chi, qigong, Pilates, or yoga

Benefits

- Fresh air
- Natural outdoor light—blue wavelength to help reduce depression
- Some sunshine for vitamin D benefits
- Sustainability—uses very little resources
- Natural aromatherapy from plants
- Principles of feng shui
- Mindfulness training:
    - Sight—see natural scenery
    - Sound—hear the birds and wind

Taste—taste the mint or basil plants from your garden around your gazebo
Touch—feel the textures of the herbs and plants around your gazebo

Possible Features

- Keep a portable massage table in a corner of your fitness gazebo.
- Install a pull-up bar to decompress your spine
- Install attachment sites for exercise elastic bands
- Install a wooden rack for dumbbells and kettlebells
- Install hooks for attaching a hammock
- Install a wood floor so you can perform tai chi, qigong, yoga, or Pilates in your private healing gazebo
- Place a rocking chair in the gazebo for sitting while drinking healing green tea
- Create a healing herb garden to surround your gazebo

Additional Labyrinth Resources

- A Maze Your Mind: Labyrinth Solutions, www.amazeyourmindlabyrinths.com
- Labyrinth Company, www.labyrinthcompany.com
- Relax4Life, www.relax4life.com
- The Labyrinth Society, http://labyrinthsociety.org
- Veriditas, www.veriditas.org

Additional Mindfulness Resources

- Benson-Henry Institute for Mind Body Medicine, www.bensonhenryinstitute.org
- Center for Investigating Healthy Minds, www.investigatinghealthyminds.org
- Center for Mindfulness in Medicine, Health Care, and Society, www.umassmed.edu/cfm
- Headspace app, www.headspace.com
- Institute for Mindful Leadership, http://instituteformindfulleadership.org
- Mind & Life Institute, www.mindandlife.org
- Mind Fitness Training Institute, www.mind-fitness-training.org
- *Mindful* magazine, www.mindful.org

- Mindfulness Apps, http://mindfulnessapps.com
- Mindfulness & Health, www.mindfulnesshealth.com
- Mindfulness in Education Network, www.mindfuled.org
- Mindful-Way Stress Reduction, http://mindful-way.com
- The Center for Contemplative Mind in Society, www.contemplativemind.org
- UCLA Mindful Awareness Research Center, http://marc.ucla.edu
- UCSD Center for Mindfulness, https://ucsdcfm.wordpress.com

References

Bhatt SP, Luqman-Arafath TK, Gupta AK, et al. (2013). Volitional pursed lips breathing in patients with stable chronic obstructive pulmonary disease improves exercise capacity. *Chronic Respiratory Disease* 10 (1): 5–10.

Bigard M. (2009). Walking the labyrinth: An innovative approach to counseling center outreach. Journal of College Counseling 12 (2): 137–148.

Chaitow L, Bradley D, and Gilbert C. (2014). *Recognizing and Treating Breathing Disorders: A Multidisciplinary Approach*, 2nd ed. New York, NY: Churchill Livingstone Elsevier.

Chen KW, Berger CC, Manheimer E, et al. (2012). Meditative therapies for reducing anxiety: A systematic review and meta-analysis of randomized controlled trials. *Depression and Anxiety* 29 (7): 545–562.

Daniels M. (2008). An intrapersonal approach to enhance student performance. Florida Communication Journal 36 (2): 89–102.

Eason, C. (2004). The Complete Guide to Labyrinths. Berkley, CA: The Crossing Press.

Eherer AJ, Netolitzky F, Hogenauer C, et al. (2012). Positive effect of abdominal breathing exercise on gastroesophageal reflux disease: A randomized, controlled study. *American Journal of Gastroenterology* 107 (3): 372–378.

Fredrickson BL, Cohn MA, Coffey KA, et al. (2008). Open hearts build lives: Positive emotions, induced through loving-kindness meditation, build consequential personal resources. *Journal of Personality and Social Psychology* 95 (5): 1045–1062.

Hong Y, and Jacinto G. (2012). Reality therapy and the labyrinth: A strategy for practice. Journal of Human Behavior in the Social Environment 22 (6): 619–634.

Jacobson E. (1962). *Progressive Relaxation*, 4th ed. Chicago, IL: University of Chicago Press.

Jacobson E. (1964). *Anxiety and Tension Control*. Philadelphia, PA: JB Lippincott.

Jacobson E. (1964). *Self-Operations Control Manual*. Chicago, IL: National Foundation for Progressive Relaxation.

Jacobson E. (1967). *Tension in Medicine.* Springfield, IL: Charles C Thomas.

Jacobson E. (1976). *You Must Relax,* 5th ed. New York, NY: McGraw-Hill Book Company, Inc.

Johnson DC, Thom NJ, Stanley EA, et al. (2014). Modifying resilience mechanisms in at-risk individuals: A controlled study of mindfulness training in Marines preparing for deployment. *American Journal of Psychiatry* 171 (8): 844–853.

Kabat-Zinn J. (2003). Mindfulness-based interventions in context: Past, present, and future. *Clinical Psychology: Science and Practice* 10: 144–56.

Kabat-Zinn J. (2005). *Wherever You Go, There You Are: Mindfulness Meditation in Everyday Life,* 10th ed. New York, NY: Hyperion.

Kabat-Zinn J. (2005). *Coming to Our Senses: Healing Ourselves and the World Through Mindfulness.* New York, NY: Hyperion.

Kabat-Zinn J. (2007). *Arriving at Your Own Door: 108 Lessons in Mindfulness.* New York, NY: Hyperion.

Kisner C, and Colby LA. (2012). *Therapeutic Exercise,* 6th ed. Philadelphia, PA: FA Davis.

Marturano J. (2014). *Finding the Space to Lead: A Practical Guide to Mindful.* New York, NY: Bloomsbury Press.

Molholt R. (2011). Roman labyrinth mosaics and the experience of motion. *Art Bulletin* 93 (3): 287–303.

Ong JC, Shapiro SL, and Manber, R. (2009). Mindfulness meditation and cognitive behavioral therapy for insomnia: A naturalistic 12-month follow-up. *Explore (NY)* 5 (1): 30–36.

Ruggles C, and Saunders NJ. (2012). Desert labyrinth: Lines, landscape and meaning at Nazca, Peru. *Antiquity* 86 (334): 1126–1140.

Simpson R, Booth J, Lawrence M, et al. (2014). Mindfulness based interventions in multiple sclerosis—A systematic review. *BMC Neurology* 14: 15

Teut M, Roesner EJ, Ortiz M, et al. (2013). Mindful walking in psychologically distressed individuals: A randomized controlled trial. *Evidence-Based Complementary and Alternative Medicine* 2013: 489856.

Venes D. (Ed.) (2013). *Taber's Cyclopedic Medical Dictionary,* 22nd ed. Philadelphia, PA: FA Davis.

Wilhelm R. (commentary by CG Jung). (1962). *The Secret of the Golden Flower: A Chinese Book of Life* (a translation). San Diego, CA: A Harvest Book.

Zucker D, and Sharma A. (2012). Labyrinth walking in corrections. Journal of Addictions Nursing 23 (1): 47–54.

PART 14

Exercise Programs

The following are some fitness programs to consider spicing up your workouts:

PROGRAM 1: PHYSICAL PROGRESSIVE RELAXATION
You can have a therapist, trainer, or friend call out the relaxation sequences, or you can record the commands to play at your desired time intervals.

- To start, breathe in and out slowly three times using diaphragmatic breathing.
- Take a deep chest breath, and then relax with two diaphragmatic breaths.
- Wrinkle up your forehead for five seconds, and then relax with two diaphragmatic breaths.
- Frown for five seconds, and then relax with two diaphragmatic breaths.
- Press your lips together for five seconds, and then relax with two diaphragmatic breaths.
- Shrug for five seconds, and then relax with two diaphragmatic breaths.
- Tighten your arm muscles for five seconds, and then relax with two diaphragmatic breaths.
- Make a fist for five seconds, and then relax with two diaphragmatic breaths.
- Tighten your abdominal muscles for five seconds, and then relax with two diaphragmatic breaths.
- Tighten your buttock muscles for five seconds, and then relax with two diaphragmatic breaths.
- Tighten your thigh muscles for five seconds, and then relax with two diaphragmatic breaths.
- Flex your toes toward you tightly for five seconds, and then relax with two diaphragmatic breaths.

- Flex your toes away from you tightly for five seconds, and then relax with two diaphragmatic breaths.
- Squeeze your toes tightly for five seconds, and then relax with two diaphragmatic breaths.
- To end, smile lightly for five seconds, and then relax with two diaphragmatic breaths.

PROGRAM 2: MENTAL PROGRESSIVE RELAXATION

You can have a therapist, trainer, or friend call out the relaxation sequences, or you can record the commands to play at your desired time intervals.

Refer to the above Program 1 for the Physical Progressive Relaxation techniques, but in this case, apply the think-only technique. In other words, instead of actually wrinkling your forehead, simply think about doing it.

PROGRAM 3: DIAPHRAGMATIC BREATHING AND SPINE DECOMPRESSION

Purpose: To relax the body and mind, and decompress the spine. Diaphragmatic breathing may be helpful for stress reduction, relaxation, pain control, lymphedema, and thoracic outlet syndrome (Kisner et al. 2012).

Positions: Supine position for relaxation and decompression, or a seated position for relaxation only.

Technique and Design:

- Start by lying on your back with knees bent to approximately 90 degrees, feet shoulder-width apart.
- Breathe in through your nose as if trying to draw in a pleasant aroma. Then, breathe out as if you want to make the flame of a candle in front of your mouth start to flicker, without blowing it out (Eherer et al. 2012).
- Once you are good at this exercise in a lying position, try it when sitting, standing, or doing gentle stretches.
- Do 1 set of 10 to 20 slow breaths for a brief relaxation period. For a more extended relaxation period and also to decompress the spine, try lying on your back with your legs either straight or elevated (supported on pillows, a bolster or cushion, or placed on a sofa or chair) for 5 to 15 minutes. May be performed daily.

Precaution: If your chest rises more than your abdomen, you might be performing the exercise incorrectly. Try again, and be patient. It takes practice and a little coordination to master this exercise.

Alternate Spine Decompression Strategies:

- Try a sidelying position with the knees bent, while hugging a pillow with your arms and placing a separate pillow between your knees (do for 5 to 15 minutes)
- Try assuming a hands-and-knees position (do for one minute)
- Try partially hanging from a pull-up bar or a doorframe, with your feet still touching the ground (do 3 sets of 10 to 15 seconds)
- Try relaxing in a pool (do for 5 to 15 minutes)
- Try reclining in a good reclining chair (do for 5 to 15 minutes)
- Try a rocking chair (do for 5 to 15 minutes)
- Speak with a medical professional about using a spine belt or brace
- Speak with a medical professional about using a traction device

PROGRAM 4: MINI-MEDITATION BREAK
Purpose: To ease your mind when you can't get to sleep, before a big test, during a stressful event, while standing in a busy line during shopping, or while in a doctor's or dentist's waiting area

Positions: Sitting or supine

Technique and Design:

- See Program 1: Diaphragmatic Breathing and Spine Decompression in the Diaphragmatic Breathing Training.
- Do 5 to 20 slow diaphragmatic breaths as you focus on pleasant scenery such as a beach or mountain overlook (or other relaxing mental images of your choice).

PROGRAM 5: MINDFULNESS WALKING PROGRAM
A study by Teut et al. (2013) indicates that a mindful walking program can help reduce psychological stress and improve quality of life.

Purpose: Mental and physical relaxation

Location: Pick a pleasant place to walk, such as a park, university campus, neighborhood, or local trail

Technique and Design:

- On a day prior to your relaxation walk, time the course you will be walking so there will be no need to look at a watch to know how long you have been walking. You can time a course for 15 minutes to an hour, depending on your fitness level and goals.
- Bring a small bottle of water flavored with some mint or basil leaves (or fruits like a cut strawberry).
- Before you start the walk, take off your watch and turn off your phone.
- Ideally, during the relaxation walking program, you should make no judgments (about yourself or others), no decisions, and no plans.
- Start walking slowly, and continue walking at a pace your body is comfortable with for the day. Some days you might walk slowly and others days faster. This is not an aerobic routine for burning calories (although some calories will be burned). This program is for relaxation.
- Check your posture as you walk. How do you carry yourself? Are you tense or relaxed? Make small adjustments, such as walk tall and relaxed with your head up, for comfort and ease of movement.
- Focus on your feet. Feel each step for hardness or softness. Make small adjustments in your walking pattern for comfort and ease of movement.
- Notice your surroundings:
  - What colors do you see?
  - What shapes do you notice in the rocks and trees?
  - How does the air smell?
  - Do you hear or see any birds and animals?
  - Do you feel the wind in your face?
  - How do your clothes feel on your body?
  - Take a small sip of your water. How does it taste?
- Notice your breathing. Is it slow or fast? Make small adjustments in your breathing pattern to see if you feel better, move freer, and breathe easier.

- Notice your thoughts. Where does your mind want to drift off to?
- At the end of your walk, stop and perform the Calf Stretch exercise (see Part 15). Instead of counting to 30, breathe in and out slowly 10 times as you stretch each leg.
- Sit or lie down in the grass. Close your eyes, and relax. Feel the texture of the surface you are sitting or lying on. Is the surface firm or soft, warm or cool?
- Take 10 to 20 diaphragmatic breaths (refer to Program 1: Diaphragmatic Breathing and Spine Decompression section). Think about a color, sound, shape, taste, or feeling you experienced during your walk as you continue breathing diaphragmatically.
- Enjoy the rest of your day.

PROGRAM 6: LABYRINTH WALKING PROGRAM

The labyrinth in an ancient meditative tool which has been in existence for thousands of years (Bigard 2009). Some of the ancient Nazca Lines in Peru may have been a labyrinth at one time for spiritual or meditation purposes (Ruggles et al. 2012). A labyrinth is unlike a maze, since you cannot get lost in a labyrinth. A walking labyrinth brings you to the center and out again (Daniels 2008). A maze is a game and is designed to make us lose our way. A labyrinth is designed to help a person find their way physically, mentally, and spiritually.

Purpose: Mental and physical relaxation. Also, a labyrinth may be used to train the vestibular system and help improve balance and coordination.

Locations:

- Find a labyrinth path in your community by checking the World-Wide Labyrinth Locator website at http://labyrinthlocator.com. A walking labyrinth may be found at public parks, schools, medical centers, rehabilitation centers, museums, or churches.
- Create your own labyrinth in your community or backyard by using stones, ropes, or a canvas.
- Create or use a paper or wood carving labyrinth for you to trace with your fingertip.
- Take a virtual labyrinth walk at https://labyrinthsociety.org/virtual-labyrinth-walk.

Technique:

- Take several diaphragmatic breaths to help clear your mind.
- Enter the labyrinth. Allow the walk or finger tracing on a paper labyrinth to take you on whatever mental and physical journey that is intended for that day.
- As you exit the labyrinth, take note of how you feel.

PROGRAM 7: HOME AEROBIC AND STRENGTH CIRCUIT

Circuit training is a training method that involves moving from one activity or exercise to the other with varying amounts of rest or stretching in between. The advantage of circuit training is that by varying the workouts, you can exercise quickly and efficiently while using many different kinds of equipment. Circuit training may be used to enhance athletic performance, work performance, and activities of daily living (Altug et al. 1990; Morgan et al. 1972). This type of training can be used for general fitness, designed to either emphasize the aerobic, strength, flexibility, or balance component of a workout.

- Start: Warm-up with mobility exercises for 5 minutes...
- Walk in your home for 5 minutes...
- Shortstop Squats for 10 repetitions...
- Walk in your home for 5 minutes...
- Elastic Rows for 10 repetitions...
- Walk in your home for 5 minutes...
- Supine Bridge for 10 repetitions...
- Walk in your home for 5 minutes...
- Elevated Push-Ups for 10 repetitions...
- Walk in your home for 5 minutes...
- Heel Raises for 10 repetitions...
- Cool-down and stretch gently for 5 minutes...
- End: Drink adequate fluids and relax

PROGRAM 8: HOME STRENGTH CIRCUIT

- Start: Warm-up with mobility exercises for 5 minutes...
- Slow March in Place for 1 minute...
- Shortstop Squats for 10 repetitions...
- Slow March in Place for 1 minute...

- Heel Raises for 10 repetitions...
- Slow March in Place for 1 minute...
- Tai Chi Steps for 1 minute...
- Slow March in Place for 1 minute...
- Kettlebell Rows for 10 repetitions...
- Slow March in Place for 1 minute...
- Elevated Push-ups for 10 repetitions...
- Slow March in Place for 1 minute...
- Supine Bridge for 10 repetitions...
- Slow March in Place for 1 minute...
- Bird Dog pose for 10 repetitions...
- Slow March in Place for 1 minute...
- Cool-down and stretch gently for 5 minutes.
- End: Drink adequate fluids and relax

PROGRAM 9: TRACK, PARK, OR NEIGHBORHOOD CIRCUIT

- Start: Warm-up with mobility exercises for 5 minutes...
- Walk outdoors for 5 minutes
- Shortstop Squats for 10 repetitions...
- Walk outdoors for 5 minutes
- Elevated Push-ups for 10 repetitions...
- Walk outdoors for 5 minutes ...
- Tai Chi Steps for 1 minute...
- Walk outdoors for 5 minutes
- Slow-Motion Walk in Place for 5 repetitions...
- Walk outdoors for 5 minutes...
- Calf Stretch gently for 30 seconds...
- Yawn Stretch gently for 15 seconds...
- Look-Over-Your-Shoulder Stretch gently for 10 seconds...
- End: Drink adequate fluids and relax

PROGRAM 10: SENIOR CIRCUIT—HOME
A 70-year-old patient of mine created the following program for herself:

- Start: Outdoor walking warm-up around the house for 5 minutes...

- Walk to the living room and perform Supine Bridging for 10 repetitions...
- Walk to the bedroom and perform Elevated Push-ups from the bed for 10 repetitions...
- Walk to the kitchen and perform Heel Raises while holding on the kitchen counter for 10 repetitions...
- Walk to the front yard and perform Posture Rollouts for 10 repetitions...
- Walk to the back yard and perform Shortstop Squats for 10 repetitions...
- Walk to the living room and perform Tai Chi Steps for 1 minute...
- Walk outdoors 10 minutes...
- Walk to the living room and perform the Yawn Stretch gently for 15 seconds...
- Stay in the living room and perform the Calf Stretch gently for 30 seconds...
- Stay in the living room and perform the Outer Hip Stretch gently for 30 seconds...
- Stay in the living room and perform the Inner Hip Stretch gently for 30 seconds...
- End: Drink adequate fluids and relax

PROGRAM 11: SENIOR CIRCUIT—MALL
An 80-year-old patient of mine created the following program for himself:

- Walk for 5 to 10 minutes around the mall...
- Perform Chair Squats from the mall bench for 10 repetitions...
- Perform Heel Raises while holding onto the back of a bench for 10 repetitions...
- Walk for 5 to 10 minutes around the mall...
- Perform Chair Squats from the mall bench for 10 repetitions...
- Perform Heel Raises while holding onto the back of a bench for 10 repetitions...
- Walk for 5 to 10 minutes around the mall...
- Perform Chair Squats from the mall bench for 10 repetitions...
- Perform Heel Raises while holding onto the back of a bench for 10 repetitions...
- Perform the Yawn Stretch gently for 2 sets of 15 seconds...
- Perform the Calf Stretch gently for 2 sets of 30 seconds...
- End: Drink adequate fluids and relax

PROGRAM 12: SENIOR CIRCUIT—FITNESS CENTER
Consider the following senior circuit-training program at your local fitness center with your fitness professional nearby for safety:

- Start: Check your blood pressure and heart rate...
- Warm-up on a recumbent bike for 5 minutes...
- Shoot some basketball for 2 minutes...
- Kick a soccer ball for 2 minutes...
- Play a table tennis game for 2 minutes...
- Perform a few tai chi poses for 2 minutes...
- Perform a few modified yoga poses for 2 minutes...
- Perform a few modified Pilates poses for 2 minutes...
- Perform Shortstop Squats for 10 repetitions...
- Perform Elastic Rows for 10 repetitions...
- Perform Tai Chi Steps for 1 minute...
- Perform Heel Raises 10 times...
- Perform the Calf Stretch gently for 30 seconds...
- Perform the Yawn Stretch gently for 15 seconds...
- Cool-down on a recumbent bike for 5 minutes...
- Check your blood pressure and heart rate...
- End: Drink adequate fluids and relax

PROGRAM 13: ADVANCED OUTDOOR NATURE TRAIL CIRCUIT
A fit 35-year-old client of mine created the following program for himself. Carry a sturdy backpack with water and energy bars, and consider using walking sticks.

- Start: Warm-up with mobility exercises for 5 minutes at the beginning of trail...
- Walk the trail for 10 minutes...
- Perform Elevated Push-ups from a boulder or log...
- Walk the trail for 5 minutes...
- Perform single arm rowing movements using a rock (approximately 10 pounds)...
- Walk the trail for 5 minutes...
- Perform single arm overhead lifts using a rock (approximately 10 pounds)...
- Walk the trail for 5 minutes...
- Perform a double arm rock lift, rock carry for 10 feet, and rock lower to the ground, and repeat this 5 times (using a rock weighing approximately 10 to 25 pounds)...
- Walk the trail for 5 minutes...

- Perform a slow, double arm Darth Vader lightsaber swing using a stick to simulate a battle scene for 1 minute to engage the core muscles...
- Walk the trail for 10 minutes...
- Perform the Squat Stretch...
- Perform the Calf Stretch...
- Perform the Yawn Stretch...
- Perform the Hands-Behind-the-Back Stretch...
- Perform the Hands-Behind-the-Neck Stretch...
- End: Drink adequate fluids and relax

PROGRAM 14: FUNCTIONAL CIRCUIT

The following is a quick program that may be applied to movements of daily life (such as getting up and down from the floor) or athletic competition (such as martial arts, wrestling, or gymnastics). You might be surprised at the difficulty of this simple workout. And, like what one of my high school coaches used to say "Don't drop to the floor like a sack of potatoes."

- Start: Warm-up with mobility exercises for 5 minutes...
- Front Get-Ups (where you start standing, assume a hands-and knees position, then a
- prone position, and finally, return to a standing position) for 5 to 10 repetitions...
- Back Get-Ups (where you start standing, sit down toward your right side, lie down flat, and sit up by partially rolling toward your right and pushing off the floor to stand up. Once standing, quickly reverse the movements to your left side) for 5 to 10 repetitions (where a right and left get-up counts as one repetition)...
- Roll Get-Ups (where you start standing, sit down toward your right side, lie down and roll to your right, and stand up rolling and pushing off from your right. Once standing, quickly reverse the movements to your left side) for 5 to 10 repetitions (where a right and left get-up counts as one repetition)...
- Cool-down and stretch for 5 minutes.
- End: Drink adequate fluids and relax

PROGRAM 15: LOW-LOAD MOTOR CONTROL CIRCUIT

The following program might help train postures and retrain optimal movement patterns (Comerford et al. 2012). These basic movements might be useful for individuals in the early stages of mechanical low-back pain (Aasa et al. 2015) and also help give a person confidence to move with daily activities. The following exercise sequence may be performed up to three times a day:

- Start: Warm-up with walking for 3 to 5 minutes...
- Perform a supine (face up) alternate leg marching for 10 repetitions...
- Perform a prone (face down) alternate leg bending and straightening for 10 repetitions...
- Perform a gentle quadruped (hands and knees) to a heel sit position for 10 repetitions...
- Perform a seated single leg straightening and bending for 10 repetitions with each leg...
- Perform the Chair Squats for 10 repetitions...
- Perform the Shortstop Squats for 10 repetitions...
- Perform a deadlift motion using a yardstick or wooden pole for 10 repetitions...
- Perform alternate overhead reaches for 10 repetitions...
- Perform a gentle tennis swing motion on the right and the left side for 10 repetitions...
- Cool-down with regular walking for 3 to 5 minutes...
- End: Drink adequate fluids and relax

PROGRAM 16: MIND AND BODY FUSION CIRCUIT
The following is a fusion of mind and body movements which might be best suited for a fitness center:

- Start: Warm-up with slow mindful walking for 5 minutes...
- Perform a tai chi routine for 5 minutes...
- Perform a qigong routine for 5 minutes...
- Perform a yoga routine for 5 minutes...
- Perform a Pilates routine for 5 minutes...
- Perform a Feldenkrais Method routine for 5 minutes...
- Perform an Alexander Technique routine for 5 minutes...
- Cool-down with mindful walking for 5 minutes...
- End: Drink adequate fluids and relax

PROGRAM 17: WEEKLY CROSS-TRAINING

Cross-training has many definitions in the sports world. It refers to applying several sports, activities, or training techniques to improve a person's performance in his or her primary sport or activity (Moran et al. 1997).

In this book, the term "cross-training" indicates a training method in which exercises and activities such as outdoor walking, upper body biking, elliptical training, stair-climbing, tai chi, dancing, tennis, circuit weight-training, aerobic dance, and calisthenics are varied during the month, week, or even in a single workout session. A classic example of cross-training is when triathlon participants train using a combination of running, biking, and swimming.

Monday: walk or run for 30 to 60 minutes
Tuesday: weight-training exercises for 30 to 60 minutes
Wednesday: dance for 30 to 60 minutes
Thursday: bike for 30 to 60 minutes
Friday: weight-training exercises for 30 to 60 minutes
Saturday: tai chi for 30 to 60 minutes
Sunday: walk or run for 30 to 60 minutes

PROGRAM 18: WEEKLY CROSS-TRAINING
Monday: walk or run for 30 to 60 minutes
Tuesday: weight-training exercises for 30 to 60 minutes
Wednesday: bike for 30 to 60 minutes
Thursday: home mobility and stretching exercises for 30 to 60 minutes
Friday: swim for 30 to 60 minutes
Saturday: weight-training exercises for 30 to 60 minutes
Sunday: walk for 30 to 60 minutes

PROGRAM 19: WEEKLY CROSS-TRAINING
Monday: Pilates for 30 to 60 minutes
Tuesday: walk for 30 to 60 minutes
Wednesday: yoga for 30 to 60 minutes
Thursday: walk for 30 to 60 minutes
Friday: weight-training exercises for 30 to 60 minutes
Saturday: tai chi for 30 to 60 minutes
Sunday: walk for 30 to 60 minutes

PROGRAM 20: SINGLE-SESSION CROSS-TRAINING
Program may range from 30 to 60 minutes
Start: Warm-up with mobility exercises, followed by...
Walk on an indoor track for 10 to 20 minutes...
Exercise on an elliptical machine for 10 to 20 minutes...
Ride a stationary bike for 10 to 20 minutes...
End: Cool-down and stretch

PROGRAM 21: WALKING INTERVAL TRAINING
Interval training is a type of training in which periods of high-intensity exercise intervals (such as fast walking, running, fast cycling, fast swimming, or fast rowing) are
alternated with low-intensity exercise intervals (such as slow walking, jogging, slow
cycling, slow swimming, or slow rowing). Or, it can be thought of as alternating between difficult and easy exercise intervals. This type of training is sometimes also
called *fartlek*, which is a Swedish word meaning "speed play."

High-intensity and low-intensity intervals are alternated for a designated amount
of cycles and for a specific amount of time. In general, interval-training programs are
performed one to two times a week, with the other days of the week focusing on other
types of training (Baechle et al. 2008). Interval training can be made less taxing by using
fewer high-intensity/low-intensity intervals, reducing the total duration of the workout, reducing the duration of the high-intensity period, or increasing the duration of
the low-intensity period. The advantages of interval training are that it can help prevent boredom, potentially reduce overuse injuries by varying the periods of high-intensity exercise and low-intensity exercise, and also help improve physical performance.

Depending on a person's level of conditioning, the fast interval could be as short
as 15 seconds or as long as two minutes, and the slow interval can be as short as
two minutes or as long as five to 10 minutes. The key is to start slowly and progress
gradually.

- Start: Warm-up with mobility exercises
- Normal-paced walk (typically slow) for 5 to 10 minutes
- Fast walk (faster than normal pace) for 1 minute
- Normal pace walk for 6 minutes
- Continue with a repetitive cycle of alternating the slow walk (6 minutes) and
  fast walk (1 minute) for a total of 15 to 45 minutes
- Cool-down and stretch
- End: Drink adequate fluids and relax

PROGRAM 22: WALKING/RUNNING INTERVAL TRAINING

- Start: Warm-up with mobility exercises...
- Warm-up with normal pace or slow walk for 5 to 10 minutes...
- Run or jog for 1 minute...
- Walk for 6 minutes...
- Continue with a repetitive cycle of alternating the walk (6 minutes) and run or jog (1 minute) for a total of 15 to 45 minutes...
- Cool-down and stretch
- End: Drink adequate fluids and relax

PROGRAM 23: RUNNING OR JOGGING/SPRINTING INTERVAL TRAINING

- Start: Warm up-with mobility exercises...
- Warm-up with normal pace or slow walk for 5 to 10 minutes...
- Run or jog 1 lap around a track...
- Sprint or run fast for 100 yards...
- Continue with a repetitive cycle of alternating the run or jog (1 lap) and a sprint or run fast (100 yards) for a total of 15 to 45 minutes...
- Cool-down and stretch
- End: Drink adequate fluids and relax

PROGRAM 24: BIKING INTERVAL TRAINING

- Start: Warm-up with mobility exercises...
- Warm-up with normal pace or slow biking for 5 to 10 minutes...
- Bike fast for 1 minute...
- Bike slow for 6 minutes...
- Continue with a repetitive cycle of alternating the slow (6 minutes) and fast (1 minute) biking for a total of 15 to 45 minutes...
- Cool-down and stretch
- End: Drink adequate fluids and relax

PROGRAM 25: AEROBIC SHORT-BOUT TRAINING
Short-bout training is a type of training in which short-duration periods of exercise are accumulated throughout the day. For some individuals, shorter bouts of training are better suited for their fitness levels (such as deconditioned individuals) or busy lifestyles. Rather

than focusing on exercising for one hour continuously, an option is to break up activity throughout the day. This removes the burden of having to carve out a big block of time in your schedule, or being physically and mentally overwhelmed by long exercise sessions.

Short-bout exercise (for example, three 10-minute bouts of exercise per day) might fit into your schedule better than one long bout of exercise (one 30-minute workout session per day) (DeBusk et al. 1990). This type of program can keep the body moving throughout the day, as well as prevent stiffness from long work commutes and prolonged sitting.

Morning: 10- or 15-minute walk before work
Midday: 10- to 15-minute walk during lunch break
Evening: 10- to 15 minute walk after work

PROGRAM 26: MOBILITY, AEROBIC, AND STRENGTH SHORT-BOUT TRAINING
Morning: 10 or 15 minutes of mobility exercises before work
Midday: 10- to 15-minute walk during lunch break
Evening: 10 or 15 minutes of mobility and strength exercises after work

PROGRAM 27: COMBINATION SHORT-BOUT TRAINING
Morning: 10 or 15 minutes of yoga before work
Midday: 10 or 15 minutes of tai chi during lunch
Evening: 10 or 15 minutes of Pilates mat exercises after work

PROGRAM 28: STATIC LOADLESS TRAINING
Purpose: This type of training is only a supplement and should not be your sole form of resistance exercise. Try these exercises after recovering from prolonged bed rest, during vacations, or just as a one- to two-week break from your regular strength routines.

Positions: Standing, sitting, and lying down

Technique:

- *Warm-up*—before starting the program, warm-up for at least 5 minutes with walking and mobility exercises for the upper and lower body.
- *Gluteal squeezes*—tense your gluteal muscles while standing or lying supine or prone.

- *Thigh squeezes*—tense your thigh muscles while standing or lying supine.
- *Shoulder blade squeezes*—tense your upper back muscles by squeezing your shoulder blades together while sitting or standing.
- *Biceps squeezes*—tense the front of your arm muscles by bending your elbows 90 degrees while sitting or standing.
- *Triceps squeezes*—tense the back of your arm muscles by straightening your elbow while sitting or standing.
- *Cool-down*—after finishing the program, cool-down for at least 5 minutes with walking and mobility exercises for the upper and lower body.

Sets and Reps:

- Perform each exercise by tensing your muscles for 5 to 10 seconds as you count out loud throughout the muscle tension portions. Only tense your muscles hard enough that you can still count out loud comfortably without experiencing any dizziness or lightheadedness. Apply and release tension slowly to prevent injuries.
- Repeat each exercise 2 to 5 times with at least a 10-second walking rest break after each muscle tension for recovery.
- Perform the exercises 2 to 3 times per week for one to two weeks. During rehabilitation, your therapist might advise you to perform these types of exercises more frequently with different sets and reps.

Precautions: Avoid tension exercises if you have high blood pressure; have a history of a stroke; have a pacemaker, migraines, or excess eye pressure; recently underwent eye surgery; have a brain or abdominal aneurysm; tend to experience dizziness spells; or think the exercise is painful.

Speak with your healthcare provider if you are in doubt about any other medical conditions. If you are recovering from surgery, do not start any of these exercises until you speak with your therapist or physician.

PROGRAM 29: DYNAMIC LOADLESS TRAINING
Purpose: This type of training is only a supplement and should not be your sole form of resistance exercise. Try these exercises after recovering from prolonged bed rest, during vacations, or just as a one- to two-week break from your regular strength routines.

Position: Standing

Technique:

- *Warm-up*—Before starting the program, warm-up for at least 5 minutes with walking and mobility exercises for the upper and lower body.
- *Tennis swing*—Think tai chi movements (slow motion) as you perform a tennis forehand and backhand swing without a racket. Tense your core, leg, and arm muscles as you slowly go through the tennis swing.
- *Golf swing*—Think tai chi movements (slow motion) as you perform a golf swing without a club. Tense your core, leg, and arm muscles as you slowly go through the golf swing.
- *Basketball shot*—Think tai chi movements (slow motion) as you perform a basketball shot from the free throw line without a ball. Tense your core, leg, and arm muscles as you slowly go through basketball shot.
- *Cool-down*—After finishing the program, cool-down for at least five minutes with walking and mobility exercises for the upper and lower body.

Sets and Reps:

- Perform each exercise by tensing your muscles for 5 to 10 seconds as you count out loud throughout the muscle tension portions. Unlike Program 1, tense your muscles very lightly so that you can still count out loud comfortably without experiencing any dizziness or lightheadedness. Apply and release tension slowly to prevent injuries.
- Repeat each exercise 2 to 5 times with at least a 10-second walking rest break after each muscle tension for recovery.
- Perform the exercises 2 to 3 times per week for one to two weeks.

PROGRAM 30: BASIC POOL CIRCUIT TRAINING
Exercising in a pool or performing aquatic therapy can be beneficial for individuals with pain, and those who are deconditioned or need to recover after injury. Aquatic fitness is a great way to improve cardiovascular fitness, flexibility, and basic strength.

Purpose: To serve as a basic fitness program

Technique:

- Start: Warm-up slowly with walking forward exercises for 5 minutes...
- Walk forward and backward at a challenging pace for 5 minutes...
- Partial squats for 1 minute...
- Standing push and pull your hands back and forth in the water for 1 minute...
- Walk forward and backward at a challenging fast pace for 5 minutes...
- Standing heel raises for 1 minute...
- Standing single-leg balance on each leg for 1 minute...
- "Jog" in the deep end of the pool using a buoyancy belt or vest for 2 minutes...
- Cool-down slowly with walking forward exercises for 5 minutes...
- Stretch your calf muscles gently for 30 seconds...
- Stretch your thigh muscles gently for 30 seconds...
- Stretch your hamstring muscles gently for 30 seconds...
- Stretch your chest muscles gently for 30 seconds...
- Stretch your back muscles gently for 30 seconds...
- End: Relax by floating in the water for 1 to 2 minutes

Duration and Intensity: This program can be performed for 30 to 45 minutes. Use hand webs for extra resistance in the water. Depending on the goals of the pool program, a person may be immersed in the water from waist level to chest level.

Precautions: Wear nonslip footwear for safety around the pool. Work out with a training partner or fitness professional for safety. Also, ideally, have a clear lap lane.

PROGRAM 31: DEEP POOL CIRCUIT TRAINING

Purpose: To serve as a basic fitness program

Equipment: Flotation vest or belt for the first eight exercises

Technique:

- Start: Warm-up slowly with walking forward and backward exercises for 5 minutes...
- Perform slow bicycling motion in the deep end for 5 minutes...
- Perform running motion in the deep end for 5 minutes...

- Perform leg open-and-close motion in the deep end for 30 seconds...
- Perform leg scissor motion in the deep end for 30 seconds...
- Perform leg open-and-close motion in the deep end for 30 seconds...
- Perform leg scissor motion in the deep end for 30 seconds...
- Perform running motion in the deep end for 5 minutes
- Perform slow bicycling motion in the deep end for 5 minutes...
- Cool-down with walking forward and backward exercises for 5 minutes...
- Stretch your calf muscles gently for 30 seconds...
- Stretch your thigh muscles gently for 30 seconds...
- Stretch your hamstring muscles gently for 30 seconds...
- Stretch your chest muscles gently for 30 seconds...
- Stretch your back muscles gently for 30 seconds...
- End: Relax by floating in the water for 1 minute

Duration and Intensity: This program can be performed for 30 to 45 minutes. Use hand webs for extra resistance in the water. Depending on the goals of the pool program, a person may be immersed in the water from waist level to chest level.

Precautions: Wear nonslip footwear for safety around the pool. Work out with a training partner or fitness professional for safety. Also, ideally, have a clear lap lane.

References

Altug Z, Hoffman JL, Slane SM, et al. (1990). Work-circuit training. *Clinical Management (Magazine of the American Physical Therapy Association)* 10 (5): 41–48.

Aasa B, Berglund L, Michaelson P, et al. (2015). Individualized low-load motor control exercises and education versus a high-load lifting exercise and education to improve activity, pain intensity, and physical performance in patients with low back pain: A randomized controlled trial. *Journal of Orthopaedicand Sports Physical Therapy.* 45 (2): 77–85.

Baechle TR, and Earle RW. (Eds.). (2008). *Essentials of Strength Training and Conditioning,* 3rd ed. Champaign IL: Human Kinetics.

Comerford M, and Mottram S. (2012). *Kinetic Control: The Management of Uncontrolled Movement.* Edinburg, United Kingdom: Elsevier Churchill Livingstone.

Daniels M. (2008). An intrapersonal approach to enhance student performance. Florida Communication Journal 36 (2): 89–102.

DeBusk RF, Stenestrand U, Sheehan M, et al. (1990). Training effects of long versus short bouts of exercise in healthy subjects. *American Journal of Cardiology* 65 (15): 1010–1013.

Eherer AJ, Netolitzky F, Hogenauer C, et al. (2012). Positive effect of abdominal breathing exercise on gastroesophageal reflux disease: A randomized, controlled study. *American Journal of Gastroenterology* 107 (3): 372–378.

Kisner C, and Colby LA. (2012). *Therapeutic Exercise,* 6th ed. Philadelphia, PA: FA Davis.

Moran GT, and McGlynn GH. (1997). *Cross-Training for Sports.* Champaign, IL: Human Kinetics.

Morgan RE, and Adamson GT. (1972). *Circuit Training,* 2nd ed. London, England: G. Bell.

Ruggles C, and Saunders NJ. (2012). Desert labyrinth: Lines, landscape and meaning at Nazca, Peru. *Antiquity* 86 (334): 1126–1140.

Teut M, Roesner EJ, Ortiz M, et al. (2013). Mindful walking in psychologically distressed individuals: A randomized controlled trial. *Evidence-Based Complementary and Alternative Medicine* 2013: 489856.

PART 15
Exercise Menu

HOME EXERCISE EQUIPMENT

Consider purchasing the following equipment for your home gym:

- Quality walking or running shoes for outdoor workouts
- A quality exercise mat (when performing mat or dumbbell exercises in your home, go barefoot or wear flat shoes)
- Dumbbells or kettlebells according to your fitness level (beginner, intermediate, or advanced)
- Elastic resistance bands according to your fitness level (beginner, intermediate, or advanced)
- Stationary bike (unless you plan to walk or hike outdoors)
- Home blood-pressure monitoring unit
- Body-weight scale

EXERCISE GUIDELINES

Use the following only as a guide to determine how long, how often, and how hard you should perform each type of activity when designing your home routines. Feel free to adjust the Sample Exercise Prescription Guidelines for Basic Fitness box to fit your needs.

Sample Exercise Prescription Guidelines For Basic Fitness			
Type of Activity	Frequency of Activity	Length of Activity	Intensity of Activity
Warm-up	before each routine	5 to 10 minutes	Gentle
Aerobic Routine	3 to 5 days per week	15 to 60 minutes	Able to talk during the activity ("talk test")
Strength Routine	2 to 3 days per week	30 to 45 minutes 2 sets of 10 to 15 reps	Able to count reps out loud, with good form and without pain
Flexibility Routine	3 to 7 days per week, or after activity	5 to 10 minutes 2 sets of 10 to 30 seconds	Able to stretch gently without pain (like a yawn)
Balance Routine	3 to 7 days per week (if needed)	5 to 10 minutes	Able to perform activity safely
Reaction Time Routine	3 to 7 days per week (if needed)	5 to 10 minutes	Able to perform activity safely
Cool-down	after each routine	5 to 10 minutes	Gentle

Note: Your healthcare provider or fitness professional may need to modify these guidelines for your specific needs. Adapted from American College of Sports Medicine. (2014). *ACSM's Guidelines for Exercise Testing and Prescription*, 9th ed. Philadelphia, PA: Wolters Kluwer Lippincott Williams & Wilkins.

WARMUP EXERCISES

A warm-up is a low-intensity large-muscle activity, such as walking or light calisthenics, performed *before* a workout for the purpose of easing you into your exercise session.

Warming up before a workout helps prevent injuries and is essential for optimal sports performance (Bishop 2003, 2003). A warm-up should range from five to 10 minutes, or longer, depending on the activity and your medical condition. The following are some facts about the benefits of warm-up exercises:

- Lack of warm-up prevents blood vessels from having adequate time to properly dilate and supply working muscles and the heart with oxygen. This can result in a rapid rise of blood pressure and possibly myocardial ischemia (Abbott 2013; Barnard et al. 1973). Myocardial ischemia is defined as "an inadequate supply of blood and oxygen to meet the metabolic demands of the heart muscle" (Venes 2013).
- It's best to ease into an exercise session. The warm-up allows your body to gradually adjust to increasing physiological, biomechanical, and bioenergetic demands placed upon it.

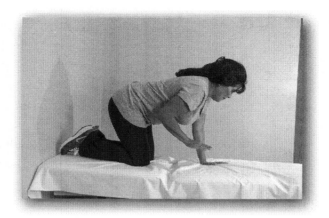

Shoulder March
Purpose: To warm up shoulder muscles
Position: On hands and knees
Technique and Design:

- Center your hands under your shoulders and knees under your hips, with hands shoulder-width apart and knees hip-width apart.
- Gently push your left hand into the floor to activate the left shoulder muscles, while raising the right hand off the floor.
- Lower your right hand, and repeat the pushing motion with your right arm.
- Continue slowly marching with your arms—think of a bear lumbering through the woods. It is considered one march when both hands move up and down.
- Do 1 set of 10 repetitions.
- This exercise may be performed daily.

Precautions: Use a soft mat or thick beach towel to cushion your knees. Skip this exercise if it causes pain in your back, neck, shoulders, wrists, or knees. Also, avoid this exercise if you have difficulty or pain getting down to the floor and back up.

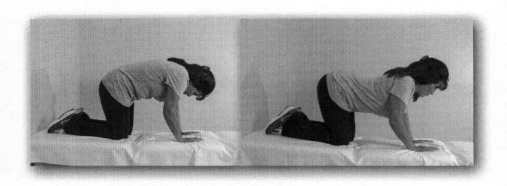

Cat/Camel
Purpose: To warm up core muscles
Position: On hands and knees
Technique and Design:

- Center your hands under your shoulders and knees under your hips, with hands shoulder-width apart and knees hip-width apart.
- Gently arch your back toward the ceiling and lower your head slightly.
- Then gently lower your abdomen toward the floor as in a scooping motion and lift your head slightly.
- Move your spine between the two midrange positions in a fluid wavelike motion.
- Do 1 set of 10 repetitions.
- This exercise may be performed daily.

Precautions: Use a soft mat or thick beach towel to cushion your knees. Skip this exercise if it causes pain in your back, neck, shoulders, wrist, or knees. Also avoid this exercise if you have difficulty or pain getting down to the floor and back up.

Additional Reading: Professor Stuart McGill, PhD indicates the cat/camel extension-flexion cycles are "intended as a motion exercise, not a stretch, so the emphasis is on motion rather than 'pushing' at the end ranges of flexion and extension" (McGill 2007).

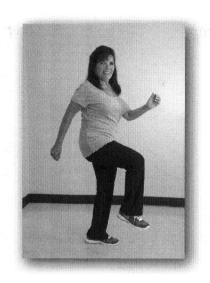

March In Place
Purpose: To warm up leg muscles, and improve coordination and balance
Position: Standing
Technique and Design:

- Start in a standing position with good posture.
- Using an alternate arm and leg motion, march in place.
- Perform 5 normal pace marches, 5 very slow marches, and then 5 fast marches. It is considered one march when both legs move up and down.
- Do 1 set of 10 repetitions, or for 1 minute.
- This exercise may be performed daily.

Progression: To increase the difficulty of the exercise, step to the right and then left, forward and then backward, and diagonally forward and then backward as you march.

Precaution: Stand near a solid object for support if you have difficulty with balance or feel unsteady.

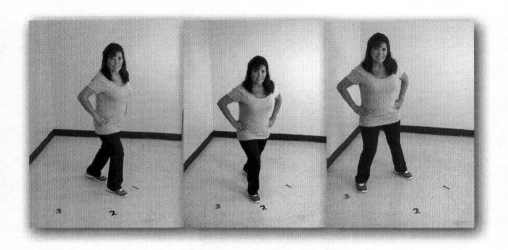

Tai Chi Steps

Purpose: To warm up leg muscles, and improve multidirectional coordination and balance

Position: Standing

Technique and Design:

- Standing with good posture, start with your hands on your hips.
- Step straight forward with your right foot (#1 position on the floor in the first photo), and return to the starting position.
- Step diagonally forward with your right foot (#2 position on the floor in the second photo), and return to the starting position.
- Step sideways with your right foot (#3 position on the floor in the third photo), and return to the starting position.
- Repeat the entire 3-step sequence with the left leg. It is considered one set when three steps are completed with the right leg and three steps with the left leg.
- Do 3 sets. No resting between sets.
- This exercise may be performed daily.

Progression: To increase the difficulty of the exercise, move both hands and arms forward (or pushing motion) and backward (or pulling motion) in rhythm (fluid motion like tai chi) with your stepping leg.

Precaution: Stand near a solid object for support if you have difficulty with balance or feel unsteady.

AEROBIC EXERCISES

There are many ways of engaging in aerobic and endurance exercises (also known as cardiorespiratory and cardiovascular fitness) such as walking, hiking, outdoor swimming, outdoor biking, or dancing, plus a variety of sports like tennis, volleyball, soccer, or basketball. Try to perform aerobic exercises at least 3 to 5 times per week. However, a basic low-intensity aerobic program, such as walking, may be performed daily.

If you have long work commutes and sit most of the day, an outdoor walk might be your simplest choice for aerobic exercise. Benefits of an outdoor walk or hike include the following:

- Fresh air
- A little sunshine, which prompts your body to produce Vitamin D (Holick 2010)
- Naturally bright outdoor light to maintain normal circadian rhythms for proper sleep and to prevent depression (Turner et al. 2008)
- Focus on distant objects for relaxation and to give your eyes a break from close-up computer work (Birnbaum 1984, 1985)
- Gentle exercise that is relatively easy on the joints (Buckwalter 2003; Kuster 2002)

If you are a member of a gym or fitness center, you can choose from an assortment of aerobic training exercises. Try a dance class, elliptical machine, recumbent bicycle, recumbent stepper, upright bicycle, stair-climber device, ladder-climber device, rowing machine, or indoor lap pool. Take advantage of all the training tools and expertise a gym or fitness center has to offer.

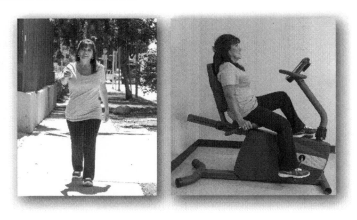

STRENGTH EXERCISES

"*Muscular strength* refers to the muscle's ability to exert force, *muscular endurance* is the muscle's ability to continue to perform successive exertions or many repetitions, and *muscular power* is the muscle's ability to exert force per unit of time," according to the American College of Sports Medicine (2014).

An article by Vezina et al. (2014) indicates that "strength training by middle-aged and older adults is critical for promoting health, functional fitness, and functional in-dependence." A properly designed strength training program is a safe and effective method for improving muscle strength and reducing weakness in elderly individuals (Aagaard et al. 2010; Coe et al. 2014). The following are practical benefits of strength exercises:

- Greater ability to get in and out of chairs with ease
- Ability to carry groceries and other items without getting injured
- Safer stair climbing
- Greater capacity to do daily chores with more ease
- Increases strength of the bones and muscles for disease prevention (such as osteoporosis and sarcopenia)
- May improve quality of sleep
- May help reduce stress

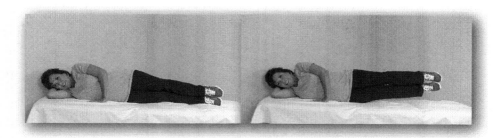

Side Leg Lift
Purpose: To strengthen the core
Position: Side-lying
Technique and Design:

- Start by lying on your right side with your right arm under your head for support. Keep your body straight through the shoulder, hip, and knees. Preserve the natural curve in your lower back and neck as you perform this exercise.
- Place your left hand on the floor in front of your chest for support.
- Slowly lift both legs together so the outside part of your right knee is approximately 1 to 2 inches off the floor.
- Hold this position for 3 to 5 seconds, and then relax for 5 to 10 seconds by lowering both legs. It is considered one repetition when both legs are raised and lowered.
- Do 1 to 3 sets of 3 repetitions. Rest 15 to 30 seconds between sets.
- This exercise may be performed 2 to 3 times per week, every other day. However, it may also be performed daily.

Progressions:

- Hold each side leg lift pose for 5 to 10 seconds.
- Do additional sets and repetitions to increase core endurance.
- Other advanced versions of this exercise include side planks. The side plank can be performed by either placing the forearm and knees on the ground, forearm and feet on the ground, or hands and feet on the ground as you lift your hip to form a straight line with your body.

Precautions: Count out loud to promote regular breathing. Use a soft mat or thick beach towel to cushion your hips. Skip this exercise if you feel pain in your back, neck, or shoulders.

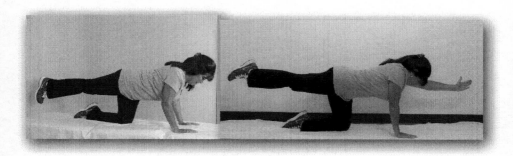

Bird Dog
Purpose: To strengthen the core
Position: Hands-and-knees
Technique and Design:

- Start in a hands-and-knees position, with your hands shoulder-width and knees hip-width apart. Find the pain-free natural curve in your lower back and neck as you perform this exercise. Stiffen your core muscles just enough to maintain your neck and back curves while still being able to breathe freely.
- Simultaneously raise your right leg and left arm, thumb pointing to the ceiling and arm approximately 3 to 5 inches away from your head, without losing your spine curve or tilting your hips.
- Slowly return to the starting position, repeating with the opposite leg and arm. It is considered one repetition when both arms and legs are raised and lowered.
- Do 1 to 3 sets of 3 to 5 repetitions. Rest 15 to 30 seconds between sets.
- This exercise may be performed 2 to 3 times per week, every other day. However, it may also be performed daily.

Alternative: This exercise may also be performed with legs or arms only.
Progressions:

- Hold each arm and leg pose for 5 to 10 seconds.
- You may also strap an ankle weight above the knee as extra resistance for strengthening the gluteus maximus muscle.

Precautions: Count out loud to promote regular breathing. Use a soft mat or thick beach towel to cushion your knees. Skip this exercise if you feel pain in your back, neck, or shoulders.

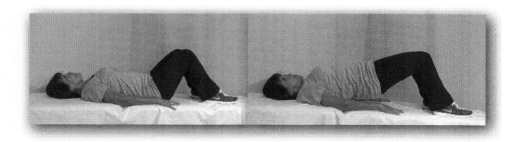

Supine Bridge
Purpose: To strengthen the hips and core
Position: Supine
Technique and Design:

- Lie on your back, with knees bent to 90 degrees.
- Moderately brace or tighten your abdominals and slightly raise your hips while preserving the natural curve in your lower back.
- Return to the starting position.
- Do 1 to 3 sets of 10 repetitions. Rest 15 to 30 seconds between sets.
- This exercise may be performed 2 to 3 times per week, every other day. However, it may also be performed daily.

Note: If you feel you are using your hamstrings and not your gluteal muscles, push your feet away from you (but still keeping them on the ground) and tilt your knees slightly outward.
Progressions:

- Hold the bridge pose for 5 to 10 seconds.
- Push your legs outward with elastic bands around your knees.

Precautions: Raising your hips too high might place a strain on your neck. Only raise your hips to where you can slide your forearm under your lower back. Count out loud to promote regular breathing. Skip this exercise if you feel pain in your back, neck, or shoulders.

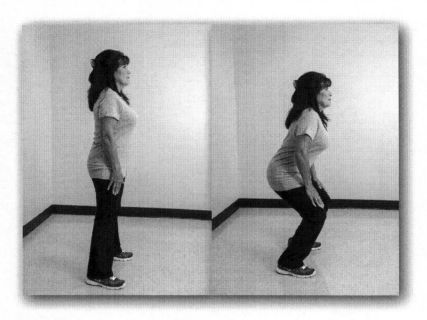

Shortstop Squats
Purpose: To strengthen legs, hips, and core
Position: Standing
Technique and Design:

- Stand with your feet shoulder-width apart and hands on the fronts of your thighs.
- Slowly bend your hips and knees as you slide both hands until your fingertips are just above your kneecaps. Be mindful of bringing your hips back and knees at or slightly behind your toes as you squat. Keep your shoulders down and back, and your knees slightly out. Preserve the natural curve in your lower back and neck as you perform this exercise. Do not squat any lower than your ability to maintain your natural lower back and neck curves. This will vary from person to person.
- Do 1 to 3 sets of 10 to 15 repetitions. Rest 15 to 30 seconds between sets.
- This exercise may be performed 2 to 3 times per week, every other day. However, it may also be performed daily.

Note: To get a little extra power, gently press your feet outward without actually rotating the feet (think of screwing the feet into the ground).

Precautions: Count out loud to promote regular breathing. Skip this exercise if you feel pain in your back, hips, or knees.

Source: Stuart McGill, PhD calls the shortstop position the "ready position" and other professionals call it the "athletic position."

Additional Information: This position is the foundation of many athletic tasks, such as waiting for a serve in tennis, baseball infielders and outfielders waiting for a batter to hit the ball, a basketball player guarding an opponent, a wrestler waiting to engage an opponent, a golfer getting ready to hit the ball, and a soccer or hockey goalie waiting for a player to shoot.

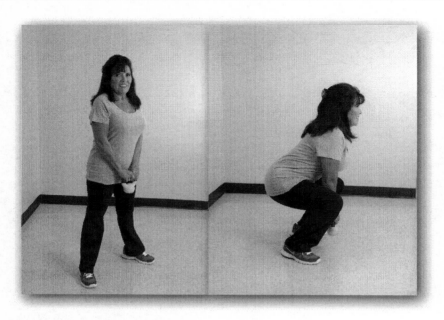

Kettlebell Floor Squat
Purpose: To strengthen legs, hips, and core
Position: Standing
Technique and Design:

- Choose a weight based on your fitness level (such as 5-, 7-, or 10-pound kettlebells for beginners).
- Stand with your feet shoulder-width apart as you hold a kettlebell close to your body with your arms straight down.
- Slowly bend your hips and knees, keeping the knees at or slightly behind your toes as you bring the kettlebell as close to the floor as possible without losing the natural curve in your lower back. As you squat, keep your shoulders down and back, and knees out. Preserve the natural curve in your lower back and neck as you perform this exercise. Do not squat any lower than your ability to maintain your natural lower back and neck curves. This will vary from person to person.
- Do 1 to 3 sets of 10 to 15 repetitions. Rest 15 to 30 seconds between sets.
- This exercise may be performed 2 to 3 times per week, every other day.

Alternative: If needed, place a 4-, 6-, or 8-inch block or pad on the floor to stop the kettlebell at a point where your lower back can no longer maintain its natural curve.

Precautions: Stop the squatting motion if you lose the curve in your lower back. Do not force the kettlebell to the floor. Have someone watch your back and give you feedback as you squat. Count out loud to promote regular breathing. Skip this exercise if you feel pain in your back, hips, or knees.

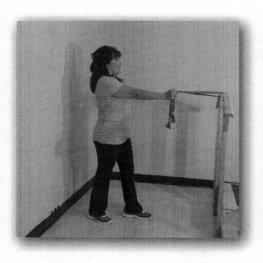 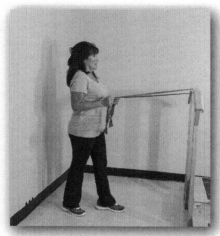

Elastic Rows
Purpose: To strengthen shoulders, upper back, and core
Position: Sitting or standing
Technique and Design:

- Start in a sitting or standing position with good posture.
- Place an elastic band around a sturdy object, such as the knob of a securely shut door or a rail, and step back just enough so the band has some tension.
- Pull or "row" the band from an arms-outstretched position to the elbows-by-your-sides position.
- Do 1 to 3 sets of 10 to 15 repetitions. Rest 15 to 30 seconds between sets.
- This exercise may be performed 2 to 3 times per week, every other day.

Precautions: Count out loud to promote regular breathing. Skip this exercise if you feel pain in your back, neck, shoulders, or arms.

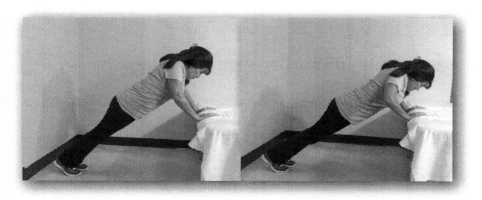

Elevated Push-Ups
Purpose: To strengthen the shoulders, chest, and arms
Position: Standing
Technique and Design:

- Stand and place your hands shoulder-width apart on a bed or other surface that is midthigh to knee height.
- Take several steps backward, placing the fronts of both feet about hip-width apart. Keep your core tight and preserve the natural curve in your lower back and neck as you bend your elbows.
- Stop when your face is approximately 6 inches from the bed, then push back to the elbows-straight position.
- Do 1 to 3 sets of 10 to 15 repetitions. Rest 15 to 30 seconds between sets.
- This exercise may be performed 2 to 3 times per week, every other day.

Precautions: Count out loud to promote regular breathing. Skip this exercise if you feel pain in your back, neck, shoulders, or arms, or have weakness that might lead to injury due to lack of control.

FLEXIBILITY EXERCISES

"*Flexibility* is the ability to move a joint through its complete range of motion," according to the American College of Sports Medicine (2014). Stretching keeps muscles and joints mobile, and it promotes ease in activities such as bending to tie your shoes or reaching the buttons at the ATM drive-thru. Stretching can be used for relaxation, correcting asymmetries, and increasing range of motion. The following are other practical benefits of stretching and flexibility exercises:

- Reduce muscle tension, pain, and mental stress
- Increase circulation
- Improve posture
- Improve function for daily tasks, such as putting on socks (hip and knee mobility) or removing your coat (shoulder mobility)

Athletes and sports participants should use caution before exercise, activity, and sports, since static stretching has been shown to acutely decrease maximal strength (Fowles et al. 2000; Winchester et al. 2009), strength endurance (Nelson et al. 2005), power (jumping) (Behm et al. 2007), sprint performance (Paradisis et al. 2014; Winchester et al. 2008), performance in short endurance bouts (Lowery et al. 2014), and provides no added benefits to dynamic stretching in terms of injury prevention in high school soccer athletes (Zakaria et al. 2015). Therefore, focusing on dynamic warm-ups before activity or sports participation, and maybe gentle static stretching *after* activity or sports participation, might be more beneficial.

The key is to avoid aggressive and prolonged stretching for general fitness purposes. Stay active throughout the day with a variety of movements, and avoid prolonged sitting or standing positions. As an alternative to stretching, you could perform the gentle movements such as basic movements such as squatting, swaying, bending, reaching, and turning.

However, keep in mind that you may need prolonged and sometimes aggressive stretching during certain rehabilitation programs (such as after knee or shoulder surgery). Your therapist will guide you in these situations.

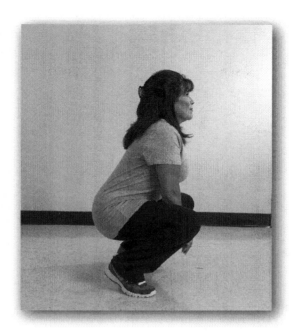

Squat Stretch
Purpose: To stretch leg and hip muscles
Position: Squatting
Technique and Design:

- Stand with your legs shoulder-width apart.
- Slowly squat down as far as you can go comfortably. Hold the gentle stretch position for 10 to 15 seconds. Stand up and relax for 5 to 10 seconds.
- Do 1 to 3 sets.
- This exercise may be performed daily.

Progression: Try keeping your heels on the ground during the stretch.

Precautions: Breathe naturally during the stretch to allow for relaxation. If needed, hold on to a sturdy object for support. Skip this exercise if you feel pain in your back, hips, knees, or ankles. Consult with your healthcare provider or physical therapist before performing this exercise if you've had total hip- or knee-replacement surgery.

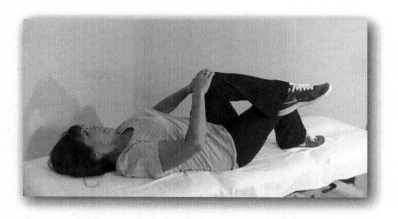

Outer Hip Stretch
Purpose: To stretch outer hip muscles
Position: Supine
Technique and Design:

- Lie on your back with both knees bent comfortably.
- Slowly bend your left hip and knee so the outer part of your left foot rests on top of your right thigh.
- Place your right hand on the outer part of your left knee, and very gently apply a force toward you until you feel a stretch in the outer left hip. Hold the gentle stretch position for 10 to 30 seconds. Relax for 5 to 10 seconds.
- Repeat with the other leg.
- Do 1 to 3 sets.
- This exercise may be performed daily.

Precautions: Use a small rolled-up towel to support the natural curve in your lower back and a small pillow under your head for support, if needed. Breathe naturally during the stretches to allow for relaxation. Skip this exercise if you feel pain in your back, hips, or knees. Consult with your healthcare provider or physical therapist before performing this exercise if you've had total hip- or knee-replacement surgery.

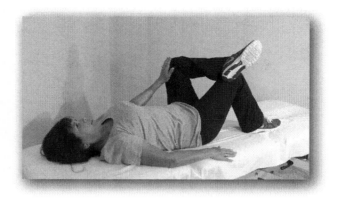

Inner Hip Stretch
Purpose: To stretch inner hip muscles
Position: Supine
Technique and Design:

- Lie on your back with both knees bent comfortably.
- Slowly bend your left hip and knee so the outer part of your left foot rests on top of your right thigh.
- Place your left hand on the inner part of your left knee, and very gently apply a force away from you until you feel a stretch in the inner left hip. Hold the gentle stretch position for 10 to 30 seconds. Relax for 5 to 10 seconds.
- Repeat with the other leg.
- Do 1 to 3 sets.
- This exercise may be performed daily.

Precautions: Use a small rolled-up towel to support the natural curve in your lower back and a small pillow under your head for support, if needed. Breathe naturally during the stretches to allow for relaxation. Skip this exercise if you feel pain in your back, hips, or knees. Consult with your healthcare provider or physical therapist before performing this exercise if you've had total hip- or knee-replacement surgery.

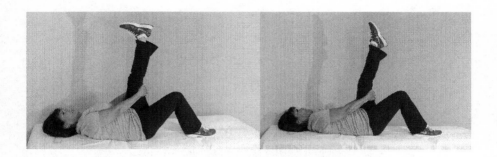

Hamstring Stretch with Ankle Pumps
Purpose: To stretch posterior thigh and calf muscles
Position: Supine
Technique and Design:

- Lie on your back with both knees bent comfortably.
- Place both hands around the back of your upper left leg and bring it toward your chest so it is at arm's length.
- Slowly straighten your left knee until you feel a gentle hamstring stretch.
- Slowly and gently pump your left ankle back and forth, flexing and straightening the foot for 10 repetitions. It is considered one repetition when the foot moves up and down one time.
- Repeat with the other leg.
- Do 1 to 3 sets.
- This exercise may be performed daily.

Alternative: If you are unable to reach the back of your upper leg comfortably, wrap a towel around your upper leg and hold the towel.

Precautions: Use a small rolled-up towel to support the natural curve in your lower back and a small pillow under your head for support, if needed. Breathe naturally during the stretches to allow for relaxation. Skip this exercise if you feel pain in your back, hips, or knees.

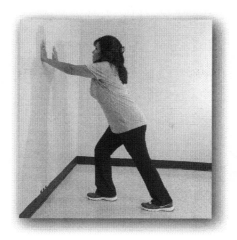

Calf Stretch
Purpose: To stretch calf muscles
Position: Standing
Technique and Design:

- Stand with your feet hip-width apart. Preserve the natural curve in your lower back and neck as you perform this exercise.
- Place both hands, at about shoulder height, on a wall in front of you.
- Position your right leg in front of you with your right knee slightly bent for support.
- Step back with your left leg, keeping your left knee straight and left foot pointed forward.
- Lean slightly with your hip and torso until you feel a gentle stretch in your left calf, heel cord, and a little in front of your right hip. Hold the gentle stretch position for 10 to 30 seconds. Relax for 5 to 10 seconds.
- Repeat with the other leg.
- Do 1 to 3 sets.
- This exercise may be performed daily.

Alternative: For variety, try turning your back foot in or out slightly as you stretch.

Precautions: You might also feel a stretch in the front of the hips, especially if they are tight. Breathe naturally during the stretches to allow for relaxation. Skip this exercise you feel pain in your back, hips, or knees.

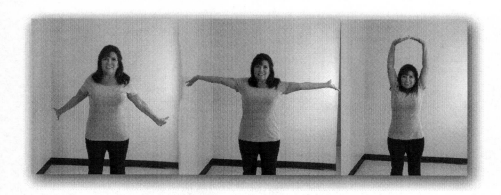

Yawn Stretch
Purpose: To stretch chest, shoulders, arms, and upper back muscles
Position: Standing
Technique and Design:

- Stand with your feet shoulder-width apart, hands by your sides, and thumbs facing forward. Preserve the natural curve in your lower back as you perform this exercise.
- Rotate your thumbs away from the sides of your body, bend your palms away from the inner part of your wrist, and draw your shoulders slightly back to feel a stretch in your forearms, shoulders, and chest (as shown in photo #1). Hold the gentle stretch position for 5 seconds.
- Bring your arms up to shoulder level, bend your palms away from the inner parts of wrists (palms facing side walls), and draw your shoulders slightly back to feel a stretch in your forearms, shoulders, and chest (as shown in photo #2). Hold the gentle stretch position for 5 seconds.
- Raise both arms overhead with your palms facing the ceiling and fingers pointing toward the middle of your body to feel a stretch in your upper back (as shown in photo #3). Finally, yawn as you stretch to relax your facial muscles. Hold the gentle stretch position for 5 seconds.
- Do 1 to 3 sets.
- This exercise may be performed multiple times throughout the day.

Note: Perform the stretch after you have been sitting for prolonged periods, such as after using the computer, watching television, reading a book, sewing or knitting, or driving.

Precautions: Breathe naturally during the stretches to allow for relaxation. Skip this exercise if you feel pain in your neck, shoulders, arms, or back.

BALANCE EXERCISES

Balance, or postural stability, is "the ability to control the center of mass within the boundaries of the base of support" (O'Sullivan 2014). Balance can be either stationary (such as holding a position in standing, sitting, or kneeling) or dynamic (such as with movement during weight shifting from one foot to another, reaching, or stepping). The following are practical areas of improvement from applying balance exercises:

- Walking on uneven surfaces, such as grass or old sidewalks
- Going up and down curbs, and climbing stairs without a rail
- Avoiding falls when somebody lightly bumps into you
- Steadily carrying a food plate
- Safely getting in and out of the bathtub
- Reduced injury during sports participation

Balance can be modified by changing feet positions, such as a narrow versus a wide stance, a tandem stance (heel-to-toe position), or a step stance (one foot in front of the other during a normal step), and by keeping your eyes open or closed. Also, balance exercises can be performed with both legs or one leg. Finally, try talking during postural stability exercises since it may optimize dynamic control (Massery et al. 2013).

Stationary balance exercises can be performed on a stable surface, such as the floor or a low balance beam. Stationary balance exercises can also be performed on an unstable surface, such as a wobble board, hard disc, soft disc, soft stepping pods, foam rubber pad, half foam roll, mini trampoline, or BOSU ball (an exercise tool that has a dome side and platform side, and stands for "both sides up").

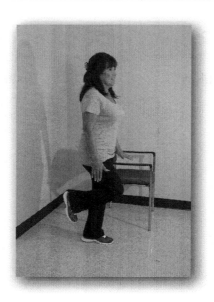

Single-Leg Stance
Purpose: To improve static balance
Position: Standing
Technique and Design:

- Stand with your feet hip-width apart near a sturdy object (such as a chair) for support. Keep your eyes open throughout the exercise.
- Slowly lift your right leg off the ground to about midcalf level, without touching your left leg. Hold this position in a safe and steady manner for 1 to 15 seconds, depending on your ability.
- Repeat on the other side.
- Do 3 to 5 sets.
- This exercise may be performed 2 to 3 times per week, every other day. However, it may also be performed daily.

Progressions: If you are able to easily stand on each leg for 30 seconds, try the following:

- Slowly swing your arms up and down like you are marching.
- Move your arms across your chest and open them out to the sides.
- Twirl a small towel in your right hand and then your left hand.

Precautions: Breathe naturally during the exercise. Skip this exercise if you experience dizziness, lightheadedness, or vertigo and report these symptoms to your healthcare provider. Also, avoid this exercise if you feel unstable and cannot maintain a safe upright posture.

References

Benefits of Warm-Up and Cooldown Exercises

Abbott AA. (2013). Cardiac arrest litigations. *ACSM's Health & Fitness Journal* 17 (1): 31–34.

Allen BA, Hannon JC, Burns RD, et al. (2014). Effect of a core conditioning intervention on tests of trunk muscular endurance in school-aged children. *Journal of Strength and Conditioning Research* 28 (7): 2063–2070.

American College of Sports Medicine. (2014). *ACSM's Resource Manual for Guidelines for Exercise Testing and Prescription*, 7th ed. Philadelphia, PA: Wolters Kluwer Lippincott Williams & Wilkins.

Andersen LL, Jay K, Andersen CH, et al. (2013). Acute effects of massage or active exercise in relieving muscle soreness: Randomized controlled trial. *Journal of Strength and Conditioning Research* 27 (12): 3352–3359.

Barnard RJ, Gardner GW, Diaco NV, et al. (1973). Cardiovascular responses to sudden strenuous exercise: Heart rate, blood pressure, and ECG. *Journal of Applied Physiology* 34: 883.

Bishop D. (2003). Warm up I: Potential mechanisms and the effects of passive warm up on exercise performance. *Sports Medicine* 33 (6): 439–454.

Bishop D. (2003). Warm up II: Performance changes following active warm up and how to structure the warm up. *Sports Medicine* 33 (7): 483–498.

Brubaker PH, and Kitzman DW. (2011). Chronotropic incompetence: Causes, consequences, and management. *Circulation* 123 (9): 1010–1020.

Dimsdale JE, Hartley LH, Guiney T, et al. (1984). Postexercise peril. Plasma catecholamines and exercise. *JAMA* 251 (5): 630–632.

Kenney WL, Wilmore JH, and Costill DL. (2012). *Physiology of Sport and Exercise*, 5th ed. Champaign, IL: Human Kinetics.

Koyama Y, Koike A, Yajima T, et al. (2000). Effects of 'cool-down' during exercise recovery on cardiopulmonary systems in patients with coronary artery disease. *Japanese Circulation Journal* 64 (3): 191–196.

Law RY, and Herbert RD. (2007). Warm-up reduces delayed onset muscle soreness but cool-down does not: A randomised controlled trial. *Australian Journal of Physiotherapy* 53 (2): 91–95.

Olsen O, Sjohaug M, van Beekvelt M, et al. (2012). The effect of warm-up and cool-down exercise on delayed onset muscle soreness in the quadriceps muscle: A randomized controlled trial. *Journal of Human Kinetics* 35: 59–68.

Paton CM, Nagelkirk PR, Coughlin AM, et al. (2004). Changes in von Willebrand factor and fibrinolysis following a post-exercise cool-down. *European Journal of Applied Physiology* 92 (3): 328–333.

Spitz MG, Kenefick RW, and Mitchell JB. (2013). The effects of elapsed time after warm-up on subsequent exercise performance in a cold environment. *Journal of Strength and Conditioning Research* 28 (5): 1351–1357.

Stickland MK, Rowe BH, Spooner CH, et al. (2012). Effect of warm-up exercise on exercise-induced bronchoconstriction. *Medicine and Science in Sports and Exercise* 44 (3): 383–391.

Takahashi T, Okada A, Hayano J, et al. (2002). Influence of cool-down exercise on autonomic control of heart rate during recovery from dynamic exercise. *Frontiers of Medical and Biological Engineering* 11 (4): 249–259.

Van Gelder LH, and Bartz SD. (2011). The effect of acute stretching on agility performance. *Journal of Strength and Conditioning Research* 25 (11): 3014–3021.

Venes D. (Ed.) (2013). *Taber's Cyclopedic Medical Dictionary*, 22nd ed. Philadelphia, PA: FA Davis.

Warm-Up and Mobility Exercises

Andersen CH, Zebis MK, Saervoll, et al. (2012). Scapular muscle activity from selected strengthening exercises performed at low and high intensities. *Journal of Strength and Conditioning Research* 26 (9): 2408–2416.

Brügger A. (2000). *Lehrbuch der Funktionellen* Störungen *des Bewegungssystems*. *[Textbook of the functional disturbances of the movement system]*. Zollikon/Benglen, Switzerland: Brügger-Verlag.

Fung V, Ho A, Shaffer J, et al. (2012). Use of Nintendo Wii Fit™ in the rehabilitation of outpatients following total knee replacement: A preliminary randomised controlled trial. *Physiotherapy* 98 (3): 183–188.

Ha SM, Kwon OY, Cynn HS, et al. (2012). Comparison of electromyographic activity of the lower trapezius and serratus anterior muscle in different arm-lifting scapular posterior tilt exercises. *Physical Therapy in Sport* 13 (4): 227–232.

Hardwick DH, Beebe JA, McDonnell MK, et al. (2006). A comparison of serratus anterior muscle activation during a wall slide exercise and other traditional exercises. *Journal of Orthopaedic & Sports Physical Therapy* 36 (12): 903–910.

Janda V, and Vávrová M. (1996). Sensory motor stimulation. In: Liebenson C. (Ed.) *Rehabilitation of the Spine: A Practitioner's Manual*. Philadelphia, PA: Lippincott Williams & Wilkins.

Kobesova A, Dzvonik J, Pavel Kolar P, et al. (2015). Effects of shoulder girdle dynamic stabilization exercise on hand muscle strength. *Isokinetics and Exercise Science* 23: 21–32.

Kurokawa D, Sano H, Nagamoto H, et al. (2014). Muscle activity pattern of the shoulder external rotators differs in adduction and abduction: An analysis using positron emission tomography. *Journal of Shoulder and Elbow Surgery* 23 (5): 658–664.

Lee S, Lee D, and Park J. (2013). The effect of hand position changes on electromyographic activity of shoulder stabilizers during push-up plus exercise on stable and unstable surfaces. *Journal of Physical Therapy Science* 25 (8): 981–984.

Ludewig PM, Hoff MS, Osowski EE, et al. (2004). Relative balance of serratus anterior and upper trapezius muscle activity during push-up exercises. *American Journal of Sports Medicine* 32 (2): 484–493.

McGill SM. (2007). *Low Back Disorders*, 2nd ed. Champaign IL: Human Kinetics.

McGill SM. (2014). *Building the Ultimate Back: From Rehabilitation to Performance* (course manual). Los Angeles, CA, April 26–27.

Morris CE, Greenman PE, Bullock MI, et al. (2006). Vladimir Janda, MD, DSc: Tribute to a master of rehabilitation. *Spine (Phila Pa 1976)* 31 (9): 1060–1064.

Moseley JB, Jobe FW, Pink M, et al. (1992). EMG analysis of the scapular muscles during a shoulder rehabilitation program. *American Journal of Sports Medicine* 20 (2):128–134.

Preisinger E, Alacamlioglu Y, Pils K, et al. (1996). Exercise therapy for osteoporosis: Results of a randomised controlled trial. *British Journal of Sports Medicine* 30 (3): 209–212.

Sahrmann SA. (2002). *Diagnosis and Treatment of Movement Impairment Syndromes*. St. Louis, MO: Mosby.

Seo SH, Jeon IH, Cho YH, et al. (2013). Surface EMG during the push-up plus exercise on a stable support or Swiss ball: Scapular stabilizer muscle exercise. *Journal of Physical Therapy Science* 25 (7): 833–837.

Shinozaki N, Sano H, Omi R, et al. (2014). Differences in muscle activities during shoulder elevation in patients with symptomatic and asymptomatic rotator cuff tears: Analysis by positron emission tomography. *Journal of Shoulder and Elbow Surgery* 23 (3): e61–67.

Yamada M, Higuchi T, Nishiguchi S, et al. (2013). Multitarget stepping program in combination with a standardized multicomponent exercise program can prevent falls in community-dwelling older adults: A randomized, controlled trial. *Journal of the American Geriatrics Society* 61 (10): 1669–1675.

Yamada M, Tanaka B, Nagai K, et al. (2011). Rhythmic stepping exercise under cognitive conditions improves fall risk factors in community-dwelling older adults: Preliminary results of a cluster-randomized controlled trial. *Aging and Mental Health* 15 (5): 647–653.

Benefits of Aerobic Exercises

American College of Sports Medicine. (2014). ACSM's *Guidelines for Exercise Testing and Prescription,* 9th ed. Philadelphia, PA: Wolters Kluwer Lippincott Williams & Wilkins.

Birnbaum MH. (1984). Nearpoint visual stress: A physiological model. *Journal of the American Optometric Association* 55 (11): 825–835.

Birnbaum MH. (1985). Nearpoint visual stress: Clinical implications. *Journal of the American Optometric Association* 56 (6): 480–490.

Carson SJ. (2013). Effects of emotional exposure on state anxiety after acute exercise. *Medicine & Science in Sports & Exercise* 45 (2): 372–378.

Chapman SB, Aslan S, Spence JS, et al. (2013). Shorter term aerobic exercise improves brain, cognition, and cardiovascular fitness in aging. *Frontiers in Aging Neuroscience* 5: 75.

Earnest CP, Johannsen NM, Swift DL, et al. (2014). Aerobic and strength training in concomitant metabolic syndrome and type 2 diabetes. *Medicine and Science in Sports and Exercise* 46 (7): 1293–1301.

Erickson KI, Raji CA, Lopez OL, et al. (2010). Physical activity predicts gray matter volume in late adulthood. The Cardiovascular Health Study. *Neurology* 75 (16): 1415–1422.

Pedersen BK, and Saltin B. (2006). Evidence for prescribing exercise as therapy in chronic disease. *Scandinavian Journal of Medicine and Science in Sports* 16 (Supplement 1): 3–63.

Aerobic Exercises

Birnbaum MH. (1984). Nearpoint visual stress: A physiological model. *Journal of the American Optometric Association* 55 (11): 825–835.

Birnbaum MH. (1985). Nearpoint visual stress: Clinical implications. *Journal of the American Optometric Association* 56 (6): 480–490.

Buckwalter JA. (2003). Sports, joint injury, and posttraumatic osteoarthritis. *Journal of Orthopaedic & Sports Physical Therapy* 33 (10): 578–588.

Holick MF. (2010). *The Vitamin D Solution: A 3-Step Strategy to Cure Our Most Common Health Problem.* New York, NY: Hudson Street Press.

Kuster MS. (2002). Exercise recommendations after total joint replacement. *Sports Medicine* 32 (7): 433–445.

Turner PL and Mainster MA. (2008). Circadian photoreception: Ageing and the eye's important role in systemic health. *British Journal of Ophthalmology* 92 (11): 1439–1444.

Benefits of Strength and Core-Strengthening Exercises

Aagaard P, Suetta C, Caserotti P, et al. (2010). Role of the nervous system in sarcopenia and muscle atrophy with aging: Strength training as a countermeasure. *Scandinavian Journal of Medicine & Sciencein Sports* 20 (1): 49–64.

Akuthota V, Ferreiro A, and Moore T. (2008). Core stability exercise principles. *Current Sports Medicine Reports* 7 (1): 39–44.

Alley JR, Mazzochi JW, Smith CJ, et al. (2015). Effects of resistance exercise timing on sleep architecture and nocturnal blood pressure. *Journal of Strength and Conditioning Research* 29 (5): 1378–1385.

American College of Sports Medicine. (2014). *ACSM's Guidelines for Exercise Testing and Prescription*, 9th ed. Philadelphia, PA: Wolters Kluwer Lippincott Williams & Wilkins.

Andersen CH, Zebis MK, Saervoll, et al. (2012). Scapular muscle activity from selected strengthening exercises performed at low and high intensities. *Journal of Strength and Conditioning Research* 26 (9): 2408–2416.

Baechle TR, and Earle RW. (Eds.). (2008). *Essentials of Strength Training and Conditioning*, 3rd ed. Champaign IL: Human Kinetics.

Biernat R, Trzaskoma Z, Trzaskoma L, et al. (2014). Rehabilitation protocol for patellar tendinopathy applied among 16- to 19-year old volleyball players. Journal of Strength and Conditioning Research 28 (1): 43–52.

Chinkulprasert C, Vachalathiti R, and Powers CM. (2011). Patellofemoral joint forces and stress during forward step-up, lateral step-up, and forward step-down exercises. *Journal of Orthopaedic & Sports Physical Therapy* 41 (4): 241–248.

Cholewicki J, McGill SM, and Norman RW. (1991). Lumbar spine loads during the lifting of extremely heavy weights. *Medicine and Science in Sports and Exercise* 23 (10): 1179–1186.

Chung E, Lee BH, and Hwang S. (2014). Core stabilization exercise with real-time feedback for chronic hemiparetic stroke: A pilot randomized controlled trials. *Restorative Neurology and Neuroscience* 32 (2): 313–321.

Clemson L, Fiatarone Singh MA, Bundy A, et al. (2012). Integration of balance and strength training into daily life activity to reduce rate of falls in older people (the life study): Randomised parallel trial. *BMJ* 345: e4547.

Coe DP, and Fiatarone Singh MA. (2014). Exercise prescription in special populations: Women, pregnancy, children, and older adults. In: Swain DP (Ed.) *ACSM's Resource Manual for Guidelines for Exercise Testing and Prescription*, 7th ed. Philadelphia, PA: Wolters Kluwer-Lippincott Williams & Wilkins.

Cormie P, Pumpa K, Galvao DA, et al. (2013). Is it safe and efficacious for women with lymphedema secondary to breast cancer to lift heavy weights during exercise: A randomised controlled trial. *Journal of Cancer Survivorship* 7 (3): 413–424.

Dusunceli Y, Ozturk C, Atamaz F, et al. (2009). Efficacy of neck stabilization exercises for neck pain: A randomized controlled study. *Journal of Rehabilitation Medicine* 41 (8): 626–631.

Earl JE, and Hoch AZ. (2011). A proximal strengthening program improves pain, function, and biomechanics in women with patellofemoral pain syndrome. *American Journal of Sports Medicine* 39 (1): 154–163.

Ekstrom RA, Donatelli RA, and Carp KC. (2007). Electromyographic analysis of core trunk, hip, and thigh muscles during 9 rehabilitation exercises. *Journal of Orthopaedic & Sports Physical Therapy* 37 (12): 754–762.

Escamilla RF, Lewis C, Bell D, et al. (2010). Core muscle activation during Swiss ball and traditional abdominal exercises. *Journal of Orthopaedic & Sports Physical Therapy* 40 (5): 265–276.

Fiatarone MA, Marks EC, Ryan ND, et al. (1990). High-intensity strength training in nonagenarians. Effects on skeletal muscle. *JAMA* 263 (22): 3029–3034.

Fiatarone MA, O'Neill EF, Ryan ND, et al. (1994). Exercise training and nutritional supplementation for physical frailty in very elderly people. *New England Journal of Medicine* 330 (25): 1769–1775.

Figuers CC. (2010). Physical therapy management of pelvic floor dysfunction. In: Irion JM, and Irion GL. *Women's Health in Physical Therapy*. Philadelphia, PA: Wolters Kluwer Lippincott Williams & Wilkins.

Guo LY, Wang YL, Huang YH, et al. (2012). Comparison of the electromyographic activation level and unilateral selectivity of erector spinae during different selected movements. *International Journal of Rehabilitation Research* 35 (4): 345–351.

Ha SM, Kwon OY, Cynn HS, et al. (2012). Comparison of electromyographic activity of the lower trapezius and serratus anterior muscle in different arm-lifting scapular posterior tilt exercises. *Physical Therapy in Sport* 13 (4): 227–232.

Hardwick DH, Beebe JA, McDonnell MK, et al. (2006). A comparison of serratus anterior muscle activation during a wall slide exercise and other traditional exercises. *Journal of Orthopaedic & Sports Physical Therapy* 36 (12): 903–910.

Hulme JA. (2002). *Pelvic Pain and Low Back Pain: A Handbook for Self-Care & Treatment.* Missoula, MT: Phoenix Publishing. http://phoenixcoresolutions.com.

Idland G, Sylliaas H, Mengshoel AM, et al. (2014). Progressive resistance training for community-dwelling women aged 90 or older: A single-subject experimental design. *Disability and Rehabilitation* 36 (15): 1240–1248.

Jang EM, Kim MH, and Oh JS. (2013). Effects of a bridging exercise with hip adduction on the EMG activities of the abdominal and hip extensor muscles in females. *Journal of Physical Therapy Science* 25 (9): 1147–1149.

Kahle N, and Tevald MA. (2014). Core muscle strengthening's improvement of balance performance in community-dwelling older adults: A pilot study. *Journal of Aging and Physical Activity* 22 (1): 65–73.

Kim MH, Kwon OY, Kim SH, et al. (2013). Comparison of muscle activities of abductor hallucis and adductor hallucis between the short foot and toe-spread-out exercises in subjects with mild hallux valgus. *Journal of Back and Musculoskeletal Rehabilitation* 26 (2): 163–168.

Lee BC, and McGill SM. (2015). Effect of long-term isometric training on core/torso stiffness. *Journal of Strength and Conditioning Research.* 29 (6): 1515–1526.

Lee IH, and Park SY. (2013). Balance improvement by strength training for the elderly. *Journal of Physical Therapy Science* 25 (12): 1591–1593.

Leetun DT, Ireland ML, Willson JD, et al. (2004). Core stability measures as risk factors for lower extremity injury in athletes. *Medicine and Science in Sports and Exercise* 36 (6): 926–934.

Liebenson C. (2007). *Rehabilitation of the Spine: A Practitioner's Manual,* 2nd ed. Philadelphia, PA: Lippincott Williams & Wilkins.

Ludewig PM, Hoff MS, Osowski EE, et al. (2004). Relative balance of serratus anterior and upper trapezius muscle activity during push-up exercises. *American Journal of Sports Medicine* 32 (2): 484–493.

Lynn SK, Padilla RA, and Tsang KK. (2012). Differences in static- and dynamic-balance task performance after 4 weeks of intrinsic-foot-muscle training: The short-foot exercise versus the towel-curl exercise. *Journal Sport Rehabilitation* 21 (4): 327–333.

Mavros Y, Kay S, Anderberg KA, et al. (2013). Changes in insulin resistance and hba1c are related to exercise-mediated changes in body composition in older adults with type 2 diabetes: Interim outcomes from the GREAT2DO trial. *Diabetes Care* 36 (8): 2372–2379.

McGill SM. (2007). *Low Back Disorders*, 2nd ed. Champaign IL: Human Kinetics.

McGill SM. (2010). Core training: Evidence translating to better performance and injury prevention. *Strength and Conditioning Journal* 32 (3): 33–46.

McGill SM. (2014). *Ultimate Back Fitness and Performance*, 5th ed. Waterloo, Ontario, Canada: Backfitpro Inc. (formerly Wabuno Publishers).

McGill SM, Karpowicz A, and Fenwick C. (2009). Ballistic abdominal exercises: Muscle activation patterns during three activities along the stability/mobility continuum. *Journal of Strength and Conditioning Research* 23 (3): 898–905.

McGill SM, Karpowicz A, and Fenwick C. (2009). Exercises for the torso performed in a standing posture: Motion and motor patterns. *Journal of Strength and Conditioning Research* 23 (2): 455–464.

McGill SM, McDermott A, and Fenwick C. (2009). Comparison of different strongman events: Trunk muscle activation and lumbar spine motion, load, and stiffness. *Journal of Strength and Conditioning Research* 23 (4): 1148–1161.

Meinhardt U, Witassek F, Petro R, et al. (2013). Strength training and physical activity in boys: A randomized trial. *Pediatrics* 132 (6): 1105–1111.

Myers TW. (2014). *Anatomy Trains: Myofascial Meridians for Manual and Movement Therapists*, 3rd ed. London, England: Churchill Livingstone Elsevier.

Nachemson AL. (1975). Toward a better understanding of low-back pain: A review of the mechanics of the lumbar disc. *Rheumatology and Rehabilitation* 14 (3): 129–143.

Nachemson AL. (1976). The lumbar spine: An orthopaedic challenge. *Spine* 1 (1): 59–71.

Nachemson AL. (1981). Disc pressure measurements. *Spine (Phila Pa 1976)* 6 (1): 93–97.

National Academy of Sports Medicine. (2010). *NASM Essentials of Corrective Exercise Training*. Baltimore, MD: Lippincott Williams & Wilkins.

National Academy of Sports Medicine. (2011). *NASM Essentials of Personal Fitness Training*, 4th ed. Baltimore, MD: Lippincott Williams & Wilkins.

National Strength and Conditioning Association. (2008). *Exercise Technique Manual for Resistance Training*, 2nd ed. Champaign, IL: Human Kinetics.

Page P, Frank CC, and Lardner R. (2010). *Assessment and Treatment of Muscle Imbalance: The Janda Approach*. Champaign IL: Human Kinetics.

Richardson C, Hodges P, and Hides J. (2004). *Therapeutic Exercise for Lumbopelvic Stabilization: A Motor Control Approach for the Treatment and Prevention of Low Back Pain*, 2nd ed. New York, NY: Churchill Livingstone.

Salo P, Ylonen-Kayra N, Hakkinen A, et al. (2012). Effects of long-term home-based exercise on health-related quality of life in patients with chronic neck pain: A randomized study with a 1-year follow-up. *Disability and Rehabilitation* 34 (23): 1971–1977.

Seo SH, Jeon IH, Cho YH, et al. (2013). Surface EMG during the push-up plus exercise on a stable support or Swiss ball: Scapular stabilizer muscle exercise. *Journal of Physical Therapy Science* 25 (7): 833–837.

Sharma A, Geovinson SG, and Singh Sandhu J. (2012). Effects of a nine-week core strengthening exercise program on vertical jump performances and static balance in volleyball players with trunk instability. *Journal of Sports Medicine and Physical Fitness* 52 (6): 606–615.

Sinaki M, Brey RH, Hughes CA, et al. (2005). Significant reduction in risk of falls and back pain in osteoporotic-kyphotic women through a spinal proprioceptive extension exercise dynamic (speed) program. *Mayo Clinic Proceedings* 80 (7): 849–855.

Tarnanen SP, Siekkinen KM, Hakkinen AH, et al. (2012). Core muscle activation during dynamic upper limb exercises in women. *Journal of Strength and Conditioning Research* 26 (12): 3217–3224.

Verkhoshansky Y, and Siff M. (2009). *Supertraining*, 6th ed. Rome, Italy: Verkhoshansky. www.verkhoshansky.com.

Vezina JW, Der Ananian CA, Greenberg E, et al. (2014). Sociodemographic correlates of meeting US Department of Health and Human Services muscle strengthening recommendations in middle-aged and older adults. *Preventing Chronic Disease* 11: E162.

Voight ML, Hoogenboom BJ, and Prentice WE. (2007). *Musculoskeletal Interventions: Techniques for Therapeutic Exercise*. New York, NY: McGraw Hill Medical.

Ylinen J, Takala EP, Nykanen M, et al. (2003). Active neck muscle training in the treatment of chronic neck pain in women: A randomized controlled trial. *JAMA* 289 (19): 2509–2516.

Yu W, An C, and Kang H. (2013). Effects of resistance exercise using Thera-band on balance of elderly adults: A randomized controlled trial. *Journal of Physical Therapy Science* 25 (11): 1471–1473.

Strength Exercises

Ahlund S, Nordgren B, Wilander EL, et al. (2013). Is home-based pelvic floor muscle training effective in treatment of urinary incontinence after birth in primiparous women? A randomized controlled trial. *Acta Obstetricia et Gynecologica Scandinavica* 92 (8): 909–915.

Altug Z. (2016). *Sustainable Fitness: A Practical Guide to Health, Healing, and Wellness*. North Charleston, SC: CreateSpace.

Altug Z. (2015). Thoracic outlet syndrome: A differential diagnosis case report. *Orthopaedic Physical Therapy Practice.* 27 (2): 112–116.

Altug Z. (2011). Energy Conservation Guide for Older Adults. *GeriNotes* (Section on Geriatrics, American Physical Therapy Association) 18 (1): 8.

Altug Z. (2010). Joint Protection Guide for Older Adults. *GeriNotes* (Section on Geriatrics, American Physical Therapy Association) 17 (5): 11.

Altug Z, Hoffman JL, and Martin JL. (Ed.) (1993). *Manual of Clinical Exercise Testing, Prescription, and Rehabilitation.* Norwalk, CT: Appleton & Lange.

Altug Z, Altug T, and Altug A. (1987). A test selection guide for assessing and evaluating athletes. *National Strength & Conditioning Association Journal* 9 (3): 62–66.

Badiuk BW, Andersen JT, and McGill SM. (2014). Exercises to activate the deeper abdominal wall muscles: The Lewit: A preliminary study. *Journal of Strength and Conditioning Research* 28 (3): 856–860.

Barton CJ, Kennedy A, Twycross-Lewis R, et al. (2014). Gluteal muscle activation during the isometric phase of squatting exercises with and without a Swiss ball. *Physical Therapy in Sport* 15 (1): 39–46.

Berry JW, Lee TS, Foley HD, et al. (2015). Resisted side-stepping: The effect of posture on hip abductor muscle activation. *Journal of Orthopaedic and Sports Physical Therapy* 45 (9):675–682.

Bo K. Pelvic floor muscle training. (2006). In: Chapple CR, Zimmern PE, Brubaker, L, et al. (Eds.). *Multidisciplinary Management of Female Pelvic Floor Disorders.* Philadelphia, PA: Churchill Livingstone Elsevier.

Bo K, Berghmans B, Morkved S, et al. (2007). Evidence-Based Physical Therapy for the Pelvic Floor: Bridging Science and Clinical Practice. New York, NY: Churchill Livingstone Elsevier.

Bo K, Talseth T, and Holme I. (1999). Single blind, randomised controlled trial of pelvic floor exercises, electrical stimulation, vaginal cones, and no treatment in management of genuine stress incontinence in women. *British Medical Journal* 318 (7182): 487–493.

Boren K, Conrey C, Le Coguic J, et al. (2011). Electromyographic analysis of gluteus medius and gluteus maximus during rehabilitation exercises. *International Journal of Sports Physical Therapy* 6 (3): 206–223.

Braekken IH, Majida M, Engh ME, et al. (2010). Can pelvic floor muscle training reverse pelvic organ prolapse and reduce prolapse symptoms? An assessor-blinded, randomized, controlled trial. *American Journal of Obstetrics and Gynecology* 203 (2): 170.e171–177.

Buatois S, Miljkovic D, Manckoundia P, et al. (2008). Five times sit to stand test is a predictor of recurrent falls in healthy community living subjects aged 65 and older. *Journal of American Geriatrics Society* 56 (8): 1575–1577.

Cambridge ED, Sidorkewicz N, Ikeda DM, et al. (2012). Progressive hip rehabilitation: The effects of resistance band placement on gluteal activation during two common exercises. *Clinical Biomechanics (Bristol, Avon)* 27 (7): 719–724.

Carriere B. (2002). *Fitness for the Pelvic Floor*. New York, NY: Georg Thieme Verlag.

Carriere B, and Feldt CM. (2006). *The Pelvic Floor*. New York, NY: Georg Thieme Verlag.

de Brito LB, Ricardo DR, de Araujo DS, et al. (2012). Ability to sit and rise from the floor as a predictor of all-cause mortality. *European Journal of Preventive Cardiology* 21 (7): 892–898.

Distefano LJ, Blackburn JT, Marshall SW, et al. (2009). Gluteal muscle activation during common therapeutic exercises. *Journal of Orthopaedic & Sports Physical Therapy* 39 (7): 532–540.

Fenwick, C, Brown SH, and McGill SM. (2009). Comparison of different rowing exercises: Trunk muscle activation and lumbar spine motion, load, and stiffness. *Journal of Strength and Conditioning Research* 23 (5): 1408–1417.

Flanagan S, Salem GJ, Wang MY, et al. (2003). Squatting exercises in older adults: Kinematic and kinetic comparisons. *Medicine and Science in Sports and Exercise* 35 (4): 635–643.

Flanagan SP, Song JE, Wang MY, et al. (2005). Biomechanics of the heel-raise exercise. *Journal of Aging Physical Activity* 13 (2): 160–171.

Garcia-Vaquero MP, Moreside JM, Brontons-Gil E, et al. (2012). Trunk muscle activation during stabilization exercises with single and double leg support. *Journal of Electromyography and Kinesiology* 22 (3): 398–406.

Guo LY, Wang YL, Huang YH, et al. (2012). Comparison of the electromyographic activation level and unilateral selectivity of erector spinae during different selected movements. *International Journal of Rehabilitation Research* 35 (4): 345–351.

Holmberg D, Grantz H, and Michaelson. (2012). Treating persistent low back pain with deadlift training: A single subject experimental design with a 15-month follow-up. *Advances in Physiotherapy* 14: 61–70.

Jang EM, Kim MH, and Oh JS. (2013). Effects of a bridging exercise with hip adduction on the EMG activities of the abdominal and hip extensor muscles in females. *Journal of Physical Therapy Science* 25 (9): 1147–1149.

Janssen WG, Bussmann HB, and Stam, H. J. (2002). Determinants of the sit-to-stand movement: A review. *Physical Therapy* 82 (9): 866–879.

Jones CJ, Rikli RE, and Beam WC. (1999). A 30-s chair stand test as a measure of lower body strength in community residing older adults. Research Quarterly for Exercise and Sport 70 (2): 113–119.

John D. (2009). Never Let Go: A Philosophy of Lifting, Living and Learning. Aptos, CA: On Target Publications.

John D. (2013). Intervention: Course Corrections for the Athlete and Trainer. Aptos, CA: On Target Publications.

Jung DY, Koh EK, and Kwon OY. (2011). Effect of foot orthoses and short-foot exercise on the cross-sectional area of the abductor hallucis muscle in subjects with pes planus: A randomized controlled trial. *Journal of Back and Musculoskeletal Rehabilitation* 24 (4): 225–231.

Kegel A. (1948). Progressive resistance exercises in the functional restoration of the perineal muscles. *American Journal of Obstetrics and Gynecology* 56: 238–249.

Kegel A. (1951). Physiologic therapy for urinary incontinence. *JAMA* 146: 915–917.

Kegel A. (1952). Sexual function of the pubococcygeus muscle. *Western Journal of Surgery Obstetrics and Gynecology* 10: 521.

Kegel A. (1956). Stress incontinence of urine in women: Physiologic treatment. *Journal of the International College of Surgeons* 25: 487–499.

Kushner AM, Brent JL, Schoenfeld BJ, et al. (2015). The back squat: Targeted training techniques to correct functional deficits and technical factors that limit performance. *Strength and Conditioning Journal* 37 (2): 13–60.

Liebenson C, and Shaughness G. (2011). The Turkish get-up. *Journal of Bodywork and Movement Therapies* 15 (1): 125–127.

MacAskill MJ, Durant TJS, and Wallace DA. (2014). Gluteal muscle activity during weightbearing and non-weightbearing exercise. *International Journal of Sports Physical Therapy* 9 (7): 907–914.

McBeth JM, Earl-Boehm JE., Cobb SC, et al. (2012). Hip muscle activity during 3 side-lying hip-strengthening exercises in distance runners. *Journal of Athletic Training* 47 (1): 15–23.

McGill SM. (2007). *Low Back Disorders*, 2nd ed. Champaign IL: Human Kinetics.

McGill SM, and Marshall LW. (2012). Kettlebell swing, snatch, and bottoms-up carry: Back and hip muscle activation, motion, and low back loads. *Journal of Strength and Conditioning Research* 26 (1): 16–27.

Moeller CR, Bliven KC, and Valier AR. (2014). Scapular muscle-activation ratios in patients with shoulder injuries during functional shoulder exercises. *Journal of Athletic Training* 49 (3): 345–355.

Moon DC, Kim K and Lee SK. (2014). Immediate effect of short-foot exercise on dynamic balance of subjects with excessively pronated feet. *Journal of Physical Therapy Science* 26 (1): 117–119.

Myer GD, Ford KR, and Hewett TE. (2004). Rationale and clinical techniques for anterior cruciate ligament injury prevention among female athletes. *Journal of Athletic Training* 39 (4): 352–364.

Noble E. (2003). *Essential Exercises for the Childbearing Year*, 4th ed. Harwich, MA: New Life Images.

Nuzik S, Lamb R, VanSant A, et al. (1986). Sit-to-stand movement pattern. A kinematic study. *Physical Therapy* 66 (11): 1708–1713.

Pelaez M, Gonzalez-Cerron S., Montejo R, et al. (2014). Pelvic floor muscle training included in a pregnancy exercise program is effective in primary prevention of urinary incontinence: A randomized controlled trial. *Neurourology and Urodynamics* 33 (1): 67–71.

Schenkman M, Berger RA, Riley PO, et al. (1990). Whole-body movements during rising to standing from sitting. *Physical Therapy* 70 (10): 638–648

Selkowitz DM, Beneck GJ, and Powers CM. (2013). Which exercises target the gluteal muscles while minimizing activation of the tensor fascia lata? Electromyographic assessment using fine-wire electrodes. *Journal of Orthopaedic & Sports Physical Therapy* 43 (2): 54–64.

Sharma G, Lobo T, and Keller L. (2014). Postnatal exercise can reverse diastasis recti. *Obstetrics and Gynecology* 123 (Supplement 1): 171s.

Sidorkewicz N, Cambridge ED, and McGill SM. (2014). Examining the effects of altering hip orientation on gluteus medius and tensor fascae latae interplay during common non-weight-bearing hip rehabilitation exercises. *Clinical Biomechanics (Bristol, Avon)* 29 (9): 971–976.

Silva P, Franco J, Gusmao A, et al. (2015). Trunk strength is associated with sit-to-stand performance in both stroke and healthy subjects. *European Journal of Physical and Rehabilitation Medicine* 51 (6): 717–724.

Souza GM, Baker LL, and Powers CM. (2001). Electromyographic activity of selected trunk muscles during dynamic spine stabilization exercises. *Archives of Physical Medicine and Rehabilitation* 82 (11): 1551–1557.

Swinton PA, Lloyd R, Keogh JW, et al. (2012). A biomechanical comparison of the traditional squat, powerlifting squat, and box squat. *Journal of Strength and Conditioning Research* 26 (7): 1805–1816.

Tarnanen SP, Siekkinen KM, Hakkinen AH, et al. (2012). Core muscle activation during dynamic upper limb exercises in women. *Journal of Strength and Conditioning Research* 26 (12): 3217–3224.

Webster KA, and Gribble PA. (2013). A comparison of electromyography of gluteus medius and maximus in subjects with and without chronic ankle instability during two functional exercises. *Physical Therapy in Sport* 14 (1): 17–22.

Benefits of Stretching Exercises

American College of Sports Medicine. (2014). *ACSM's Guidelines for Exercise Testing and Prescription*, 9th ed. Philadelphia, PA: Wolters Kluwer Lippincott Williams & Wilkins.

Avolio AP, Deng FQ, Li, WQ, et al. (1985). Effects of aging on arterial distensibility in populations with high and low prevalence of hypertension: Comparison between urban and rural communities in china. *Circulation* 71 (2): 202–210.

Behm DG, and Kibele A. (2007). Effects of differing intensities of static stretching on jump performance. *European Journal of Applied Physiology* 101 (5): 587–594.

Cortez-Cooper MY, Anton MM, Devan AE, et al. (2008). The effects of strength training on central arterial compliance in middle-aged and older adults. *European Journal of Cardiovascular Prevention and Rehabilitation* 15 (2): 149–155.

Cristopoliski F, Barela JA, Leite N, et al. (2009). Stretching exercise program improves gait in the elderly. *Gerontology* 55 (6): 614–620.

Fowles JR, Sale DG, and MacDougall JD. (2000). Reduced strength after passive stretch of the human plantar flexors. *Journal of Applied Physiology (1985)* 89 (3): 1179–1188.

Kokkonen J, Nelson AG, Tarawhiti T, et al. (2010). Early-phase resistance training strength gains in novice lifters are enhanced by doing static stretching. *Journal of Strength and Conditioning Research* 24 (2): 502–506.

Lowery RP, Joy JM, Brown, LE, et al. (2014). Effects of static stretching on 1-mile uphill run performance. *Journal of Strength and Conditioning Research* 28 (1): 161–167.

Nelson AG, Kokkonen J, and Arnall DA. (2005). Acute muscle stretching inhibits muscle strength endurance performance. *Journal of Strength and Conditioning Research* 19 (2): 338–343.

Nelson AG, Kokkonen J, Winchester JB, et al. (2012). 10-week stretching program increases strength in the contralateral muscle. *Journal of Strength and Conditioning Research* 26 (3): 832–836.

Paradisis GP, Pappas PT, Theodorou AS, et al. (2014). Effects of static and dynamic stretching on sprint and jump performance in boys and girls. *Journal of Strength and Conditioning Research* 28 (1): 154–160.

Winchester JB, Nelson AG, and Kokkonen J. (2009). A single 30-s stretch is sufficient to inhibit maximal voluntary strength. *Research Quarterly for Exercise and Sport* 80 (2): 257–261.

Winchester JB, Nelson AG, Landin D, et al. (2008). Static stretching impairs sprint performance in collegiate track and field athletes. *Journal of Strength and Conditioning Research* 22 (1): 13–19.

Wong A, and Figueroa A. (2014). Eight weeks of stretching training reduces aortic wave reflection magnitude and blood pressure in obese postmenopausal women. *Journal of Human Hypertension* 28 (4): 246–250.

Yamamoto K, Kawano H, Gando Y, et al. (2009). Poor trunk flexibility is associated with arterial stiffening. *American Journal of Physiology. Heart and Circulatory Physiology* 297 (4): H1314–1318.

Zakaria AA, Kiningham RB, and Sen A. (2015). The effects of static and dynamic stretching on injury prevention in high school soccer athletes. A randomized trial. *Journal of Sport Rehabilitation* 24 (3):229–235.

Stretching Exercises

American College of Sports Medicine. (2014). *ACSM's Guidelines for Exercise Testing and Prescription*, 9th ed. Philadelphia, PA: Wolters Kluwer Lippincott Williams & Wilkins.

Hartmann H, Wirth K, and Klusemann M. (2013). Analysis of the load on the knee joint and vertebral column with changes in squatting depth and weight load. *Sports Medicine* 43 (10): 993–1008.

Lamontagne M, Kennedy MJ, and Beaule PE. (2009). The effect of cam FAI on hip and pelvic motion during maximum squat. *Clinical Orthopaedics and Related Research* 467 (3): 645–650.

Winters MV, Blake CG, Trost JS et al. (2004). Passive versus active stretching of hip flexor muscles in subjects with limited hip extension: A randomized clinical trial. *Physical Therapy* 84 (9): 800–807.

Benefits of Balance Exercises

Bieryla KA, and Dold NM. (2013). Feasibility of Wii Fit training to improve clinical measures of balance in older adults. *Clinical Interventions in Aging* 8: 775–781.

Furman JM, Cass SP, and Whitney SL. (2010). *Vestibular Disorders: A Case Study Approach to Diagnosis and Treatment*, 3rd ed. New York, NY: Oxford University Press.

Herdman SJ. (2007). *Vestibular Rehabilitation*, 3rd ed. Philadelphia, PA: FA Davis.

Hirase T, Inokuchi S, Matsusaka N, et al. (2015). Effects of a balance training program using a foam rubber pad in community-based older adults: A randomized controlled trial. *Journal of Geriatric Physical Therapy* 38 (2): 62–70.

Lee S, Park J, and Lee D. (2013). Effects of an exercise program using aero-step equipment on the balance ability of normal adults. *Journal of Physical Therapy Science* 25 (8): 937–940.

Liao CD, Liou TH, Huang YY, et al. (2013). Effects of balance training on functional outcome after total knee replacement in patients with knee osteoarthritis: A randomized controlled trial. *Clinical Rehabilitation* 27 (8): 697–709.

Madureira MM, Takayama L, Gallinaro AL, et al. (2007). Balance training program is highly effective in improving functional status and reducing the risk of falls in elderly women with osteoporosis: A randomized controlled trial. *Osteoporosis International* 18 (4): 419–425.

Massery M, Hagins M, Stafford R, et al. (2013). Effect of airway control by glottal structures on postural stability. *Journal of Applied Physiology (1985)* 115 (4): 483–490. www.masserypt.com.

Ogaya S, Ikezoe T, Soda N, et al. (2011). Effects of balance training using wobble boards in the elderly. *Journal of Strength and Conditioning Research* 25 (9): 2616–2622.

O'Sullivan SB, Schmitz TJ, and Fulk GD. (2014). *Physical Rehabilitation*, 6th ed. Philadelphia, PA: FA Davis Company.

PART 16
Tracking your Progress

Have you ever wondered, "Why do I hurt all over today?" or "Why don't I have any energy this week?" or "How come I haven't lost this extra weight?" It all goes back to what my physician father once said: "How you feel is rarely a random event." Many aspects of our health are not random. Our health is a mainly a result of habits, choices, and environment.

A practical way to establish daily focus on good health before tackling any other tasks is to ask yourself these five questions first thing every morning:

- "What will I eat today for meals and snacks?"
- "What type of physical exercise am I going to do?"
- "What am I going to do for fun?"
- "What are today's personal goals?"
- "What time am I going to sleep tonight?"

A personal diary is an important tool you can use to track habits and goals. Your diary can help guide you as you lose and maintain weight, get in shape, monitor and figure out dietary intake and chronic pain (if pain is present), and also log sleep patterns. Once you know which habits are beneficial to you, you'll be able to better incorporate them into your lifestyle. A diary also encourages you to develop discipline and make the most of each day. Write in a small journal book (Altug 2011), on a paper calendar (Altug 2011), electronic calendar (such as one on a computer, smartphone, or tablet) (Hutchesson et al. 2015), or a personal blog. Use your personal diary to track any of the following:

Workouts
Track strength, aerobics, and flexibility.
Sample entry: "Exercise—Monday walk x 60 minutes"

Daily Diet
Keep track of all foods to encourage healthfully balanced eating and prevent overeating. You can also use your journal to note any food sensitivities or allergies.
Sample entry: "Breakfast—two eggs, two slices of bread with honey, one orange, water—8:00 a.m."

Daily Supplements
Keeping track of the brands, amounts, and times of any supplements you take can help you and your physician figure out if they are effective, causing you discomfort, or interfering with other medications. For instance, calcium supplements should *not* be taken with thyroid medications (such as Synthroid) because they affect the absorption of your medication, making it less effective.
Sample entry: "Supplement—calcium 500 mg—12:30 p.m."

Weight Loss
Track weekly weight loss, taking note of how certain activities and habits coincide with changes in your body weight.
Sample entry: "Weight—135 pounds—Sunday, two pounds lost since last weighed on Thursday"

Sleep Pattern
Keep a log of sleep patterns and compare to certain foods and activities noted in your journal. For example, perhaps you'll notice that you experienced insomnia the same night you swigged an after-dinner double cappuccino.
Sample entry: "Sleep—10:00 p.m.–6:00 a.m. = eight hours uninterrupted"

Stress Level
Record daily stress levels to pinpoint triggers. Use a numeric scale of zero to 10 for gauging stress: zero represents no stress, five is moderate stress, and 10 is the worst possible stress. For example, a high level of stress right around rush hour could mean it's time to find a solution to your long, hectic commute. Change your route, or join a van pool.
Sample entry: "Stress level—eight out of 10—5:00 p.m."

Pain Level

Make note of pain and symptoms related to headaches, fibromyalgia, neck pain, and back pain. By tracking your pain along with your diet, exercise, sleep, and stress levels, you might notice patterns. For example, if you're regularly waking up in the morning with pain, it might be time to get a new mattress. It also helps you better describe symptoms to your physician. Incorporate a pain scale, similar to the stress scale noted above, with zero being no pain, five as moderate pain, and 10 the worst possible pain.

Sample entry: "Lower-back pain—six out of 10—5:00 a.m."

Blood Sugar

Keep track of your blood sugar if you are diabetic. Again, watch for patterns. For example, take notice if your blood sugar is off-kilter before breakfast.

Sample entry: "Sugar—105 mg/dL—7:30 a.m."

Blood Pressure

Keep track of your blood pressure if you have hypertension.

Sample entry: "Blood Pressure—130/80—7:30 a.m."

Medications

Keep track of your medications. Many medications need to be taken consistently at the same time so they are effective.

Sample entry: "Medication—Synthroid, 50 mcg—6:00 a.m."

Home Rehabilitation

Track the progress of your physical therapy (PT) or home rehabilitation exercise program.

Sample entry: "PT—10 minutes—10:00 a.m."

Personal Thoughts

Keep track of any personal thoughts, dreams, and goals to make them real. Each day matters. Or keep track of emotions and frustrations as a way to release and relieve stress.

Sample entry: "Tomorrow I ask for a raise" or "Today I got my raise!" or "First day of my European vacation" or "I will reassess my skill set to see what I can improve upon for a future job opportunity."

Sample Journal Formats

The following sample daily journal box shows an example of a diary format you can create either in a paper journal or on an electronic blog:

Sample Daily Journal

Date:
January 1, 2017

Exercise:
Walk x 30 minutes
Yoga x 15 minutes

Nutrition:
Breakfast—bowl of oatmeal with blueberries, nuts, and honey, one cup yogurt, one cup tea
Lunch—turkey-and-vegetable sandwich, one banana, one cup yogurt, two cups water
Dinner—six-ounce salmon steak, large salad, one pear, two cups water
Snacks—water throughout day, nuts

Diary:
I had a great day today. Tomorrow night I'm going dancing.

Sample and Blank Fitness Calendars

Track your home fitness program, body weight, and goals by using the following calendar samples. The first outline is a suggested way for you to fill in the various spaces.

The second is blank so you can copy or scan for personal use. Write in the month and corresponding days, and then complete the body weight, exercises, and goals sections as you progress with your fitness program.

Sample Fitness Calendar						
May 2017						
SUN	MON	TUES	WED	THURS	FRI	SAT
	1 A.M. Walk x 30 min P.M. Walk x 30 min	2 Walk x 30 min	3 Weights X 30 min	4 Tai chi x 30 min	5 A.M. Walk x 30 min P.M. Walk x 30 min	6 Weights X 30 min
My Diary: My goal for this week is to add some weight training.						
7 Tai chi x 30 min BW: 140	8 A.M. Walk x 30 min P.M. Walk x 30 min	9 Walk x 30 min	10 Weights X 30 min	11 Tai chi x 30 min	12 A.M. Walk x 30 min P.M. Walk x 30 min	13 Weights X 30 min
My Diary: I lost two pounds this week by exercising and by consuming no soft drinks.						
14 Tai chi x 30 min BW: 138	15 A.M. Walk x 30 min P.M. Walk x 30 min	16 Walk x 30 min	17 Weights X 30 min	18 Tai chi x 30 min	19 A.M. Walk x 30 min P.M. Walk x 30 min	20 Weights X 30 min
My Diary: My energy level was excellent.						
21 Tai chi x 30 min BW: 136	22 A.M. Walk x 30 min P.M. Walk x 30 min	23 Walk x 30 min	24 Weights X 30 min	25 Tai chi x 30 min	26 A.M. Walk x 30 min P.M. Walk x 30 min	27 Weights X 30 min
My Diary: My goal for this week is to drink more water.						
28 Tai chi x 30 min BW: 134	29 A.M. Walk x 30 min P.M. Walk x 30 min					
My Diary: This month I lost six pounds!						

BW = body weight in pounds
Note: Modify the program for your needs and replace activities based on your interests.

Fitness Calendar

SUN	MON	TUES	WED	THURS	FRI	SAT
☐ BW:	☐	☐	☐	☐	☐	☐

My Diary:

SUN	MON	TUES	WED	THURS	FRI	SAT
☐ BW:	☐	☐	☐	☐	☐	☐

My Diary:

SUN	MON	TUES	WED	THURS	FRI	SAT
☐ BW:	☐	☐	☐	☐	☐	☐

My Diary:

SUN	MON	TUES	WED	THURS	FRI	SAT
☐ BW:	☐	☐	☐	☐	☐	☐

My Diary:

SUN	MON	TUES	WED	THURS	FRI	SAT
☐ BW:	☐	☐	☐	☐	☐	☐

My Diary:

BW = body weight in pounds

Additional Resources

- SuperTracker, www.supertracker.usda.gov

References

Altug Z. (2011). *2012 Healthy Lifestyle Engagement Calendar*. Indianapolis, IN: TF Publishing.

Altug Z. (2011). *2012 Healthy Lifestyle Wall Calendar*. Indianapolis, IN: TF Publishing.

Anderson CM, and MacCurdy MM. (1999). *Writing and Healing: Toward an Informed Practice*. Urbana, IL: National Council of Teachers of English.

Bassett D. (2010). Assessment of physical activity. In: *ACSM's Resource Manual for Guidelines for Exercise Testing and Prescription*, 6th ed. American College of Sports Medicine. Philadelphia, PA: Wolters Kluwer Lippincott Williams & Wilkins.

DeSalvo L. (1999). *Writing as a Way of Healing: How Telling Our Stories Transforms Our Lives*. Boston, MA: Beacon Press.

Hollis JF, Gullion CM, Stevens VJ, et al. (2008). Weight loss during the intensive intervention phase of the weight-loss maintenance trial. *American Journal of Preventive Medicine* 35 (2): 118–126.

Hutchesson MJ, Rollo ME, Callister R, et al. (2015). Self-monitoring of dietary intake by young women: Online food records completed on computer or smartphone are as accurate as paper-based food records but more acceptable. *Journal of the Academy of Nutrition and Dietetics* 115 (1): 87–94.

Pennebaker JW. (2004). *Writing to Heal: A Guided Journal for Recovering from Trauma & Emotional Upheaval*. Oakland, CA: New Harbinger Publications, Inc.

Petrie KJ, Fontanilla I, Thomas MG, et al. (2004). Effect of written emotional expression on immune function in patients with human immunodeficiency virus infection: A randomized trial. *Psychosomatic Medicine* 66 (2): 272–275.

Schaefer EM. (2008). *Writing through the Darkness: Easing Your Depression with Paper and Pen*. Berkeley, CA: Celestial Arts.

Shay LE, Seibert D, Watts D, et al. (2009). Adherence and weight loss outcomes associated with food-exercise diary preference in a military weight management program. *Eating Behaviors* 10 (4): 220–227.

Index

Made in the USA
San Bernardino, CA
18 September 2017